T...
THE NEW ... CONTROL PROGRAM?

- It is completely safe and reliable, with no harmful side effects to the body.

- It helps show couples how to either plan for or avoid a pregnancy.

- It allows couples to become aware of their combined fertility potential.

- It enhances mutual cooperation, heightens sexual communication, and helps bring couples closer together.

**THE NEW BIRTH CONTROL PROGRAM
A COMPLETE GUIDE
TO NATURAL FAMILY PLANNING**

THE NEW BIRTH CONTROL PROGRAM

by
CHRISTINE GARFINK, R.N.
and
HANK PIZER, P.A.

Introduction by
JAMES P. FURLONG, M.D.

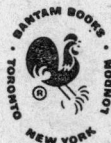

Bantam Books
TORONTO · NEW YORK · LONDON

THE NEW BIRTH CONTROL PROGRAM
*A Bantam Book / published by arrangement with
Bolder Books*

🚩

PRINTING HISTORY
Bolder Books edition published October 1977
Bantam edition / February 1979

ISBN 0–553–12567–2

Published simultaneously in the United States and Canada

*Bantam Books are published by Bantam Books, Inc. Its trade-
mark, consisting of the words "Bantam Books" and the por-
trayal of a bantam, is Registered in U.S. Patent and Trademark
Office and in other countries. Marca Registrada. Bantam
Books, Inc., 666 Fifth Avenue, New York, New York 10019.*

PRINTED IN THE UNITED STATES OF AMERICA

To our families and friends,
to their good health
and happiness

We would like to thank the people who helped us work on this book. They include all those people we interviewed; the Family Life Information Center in Albany, New York; Jeffrey Fogel and the Law Office in Newark; Paula Reich and the University Without Walls; and Alan Rinzler at Bolder Books.

Contents

Introduction

The New Birth Control Program is an idea whose time has come.

As a teacher it is always rewarding for me to see concepts take root and grow in a student. One of the authors took our early course in natural family planning taught by the Family Life Information Center at St. Peter's Hospital in Albany, New York. This present work is the result of her living with and reading a great deal about the principles involved in natural living. It is, therefore, with great pleasure that I introduce this work for better living.

The New Birth Control Program goes far beyond being a method of contraception control. It is an ecological way of life in which a couple can not only control the number of children they conceive but also their spacing—in a *natural way*.

There are no untoward side effects; no inner pollution of either mind or body. This method allows couples to live with their sexuality and to understand how mood and physical changes coordinate throughout the ovulatory cycle. And for the first time ovulation is recognized as the most important event in the cycle.

The New Birth Control Program is a simple, economical, effective, safe, morally acceptable and completely reversible way of living. This book is a clear, concise overview of the principles necessary to understand and to practice such natural conception control.

James. P. Furlong, M.D.

CHAPTER ONE

How We Got Interested

The NEW BIRTH CONTROL PROGRAM is a method for controlling fertility and pregnancy in a natural way. For this reason it has become known as Natural Family Planning. It is based on a few simple observations that when made every day, will tell a woman if she is able to conceive (fertile) or not (infertile). These observations are so simple and inexpensive that many woman can learn to use this method and practice it successfully. It is also natural in that it does not involve any chemicals or devices that invade the body and cause harm. In fact, this method is so simple that it has been used successfully in such diverse parts of the world as a modern Western city like New York and the unindustrialized, unsophisticated Pacific island of Tonga.

We began to use this new birth control method about three years ago. Chris is a Registered Nurse who was personally dissatisfied with the available methods of contraception and wanted to find an alternative. Moreover, in her work in a birth control clinic she had become aware of the increasing number of women who want to find a good alternative to the pill, IUD and diaphragm. Hank is a Physician's Assistant who studied at a teaching hospital. He became interested in Natural Family Planning through Chris, and was able to use the medical environment to study the scientific and medical literature behind the method. We have used the method together, and have found many friends and acquaintances to be enthusiastic about this new approach to birth control. So when a publisher encouraged us to write a book we felt that it would be a good opportunity to explain what we believed to be a safe, reliable, inexpensive and emotionally satisfying new form of birth control.

What Is Natural Family Planning?
Natural Family Planning is a method of birth control that allows you to choose when you want to have children and when you want to prevent conception.

This book is a simple "HOW TO" guide for people with little medical education who want to learn to use Natural Family Planning as a method of birth control. We would like the reader to kindle her/his interest by actually diving into the DOING of the method. And, after learning the simple mechanics of the program, to then go on to understand its scientific foundations. To some this may seem backwards. In most traditional learning situations we are accustomed to studying the basic foundations first, and then their applications. However, we think that anyone who is interested in finding a new method of birth control is likely to first ask, "How do I do it?", and then later want to know how it works and how reliable it will be.

The book is divided into three sections.
1. **Learning how to use the method,** so that you can determine when you want to have children and when you want to prevent conception. This is done by following the natural biological rhythms of a woman's body.

Changes are monitored by charting body temperatures taken with a mouth thermometer, and simple observations of the woman's anatomy. Together these observations can determine when unprotected sexual intercourse is safe and when it is likely to result in pregnancy.

2. **The basic anatomy and physiology of a woman of childbearing age.** This part explains why the method works.

3. **The psychology of Natural Family Planning and birth control in general.** Since the success of natural birth control depends on the emotions of the women and men who attempt to to use it, this section includes interviews with people who are using this new birth control program. In many ways this is the most interesting part of the book. These interviews illustrate the real life application of Natural Family Planning and give the prospective user an idea of how people live with the method. Because the success of Natural Family Planning depends on the total experience of women and their partners, these interviews will help you decide if the method is right for you.

All of these accounts were obtained from real people, and were recorded in live interviews. These people provide a fascinating sample of the different types of people who have found this new birth control method to be a significant advance over the pill or IUD. Many of them have rejected other birth control methods and rely entirely upon a natural form of contraception. We think that their stories are fascinating in their diversity of experience. If you like personal accounts of real people, try beginning with these stories and see if their experience with contraception is similar to yours.

How Does Natural Family Planning Work?
Natural Family Planning means following the basic fertility cycle of women. As most of us know, the physically mature woman of childbearing age is fertile somewhere in the middle of her monthly cycle. (As a point of definition, consider the first day of menstrual bleeding as the beginning of the menstrual cycle.) By avoiding unprotected sexual intercourse during the fer-

tile time, Natural Family Planning becomes a way to control when a woman and a man will have children. There are two ways to follow the fertility cycle.

1. By observing the changes in a woman's anatomy and vaginal secretions (mucus). If this secretion is present the woman is "wet" and likely to be fertile (able to conceive a child). If she is "dry" she is infertile and unable to conceive.

These secretions tell the woman when it is safe to have unprotected intercourse from the end of her menstrual period to somewhere towards midcycle. These secretions and the female anatomy itself tell a woman when to stop having intercourse.

2. By using the temperature method to determine when it is safe to RESUME having intercourse. The temperature method is a simple way to find out when the fertility period has ended for a particular month. It is used in the latter part of the cycle to know when it is again safe to have intercourse after the midcycle fertile period. (See Figure 1).

The fertility cycle of women can be divided into three parts: an early prefertile (preovulation) time, a fertile time (ovulation) and an infertile period after ovulation (postovulation). Looking at the diagram in Figure 1 you can see that we use the mucus secretions ("wet" or "dry") and anatomy in the first part of the cycle to

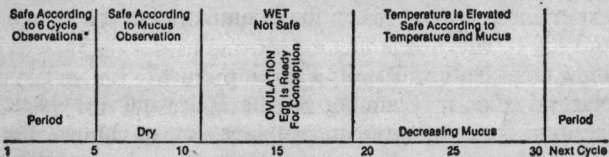

Safe According to 6 Cycle Observations*	Safe According to Mucus Observation	WET Not Safe	Temperature is Elevated Safe According to Temperature and Mucus	
Period	Dry	OVULATION Egg is Ready For Conception	Decreasing Mucus	Period
1	5 10	15	20 25	30 Next Cycle

Figure I Finding the safe days in a woman's menstrual cycle.

*For most women intercourse is safe during the menstrual period. The two conditions or situations when this is not true will be discussed in Chapter Five.

determine when to STOP HAVING UNPRO-
TECTED INTERCOURSE. The temperature method
is used to know when to START HAVING INTER-
COURSE once the fertile (ovulation) time has passed.
In actuality, both methods act as a check on each
other and are valuable through the cycle.

From Figure 1 you can see that for an average
woman with a 30-day cycle, eight days around the
middle of the month will be unsafe for having unprotected intercourse. However, each woman is an individual and must chart her own body changes. Even if
your cycle is 30 days, as in Figure 1, you may be
fertile during a different part of the month than shown
in the chart. To be used properly, Natural Family Planning involves following your own cycle, every day of
every month.

How women and men relate to the unsafe (fertile)
time is a very important part of this new birth control
program. Complete abstinence from all forms of love
making during this period often puts a heavy strain on
relationships. We think that the abstinence time can be
a period when alternate forms of loving and love
making can be employed if the couple feels comfortable
with them. For many couples this new concept provides a whole new area of growth and communication.

What is essential is that unprotected intercourse
(male penetration) during the unsafe time is almost
assuredly going to result in an unplanned pregnancy
and the failure of the method. If one uses a diaphragm
and/or condom during this time there is also an element of risk. However, the risk in this case is not much
different from using these methods on a regular basis
without regard to the natural fertility of women. We
have found in our investigation and in our personal
experience that the way people relate to the unsafe
time is very likely to be the determining factor in the
success of the method.

In summary, this new birth control program will

teach you two simple and virtually costless ways to
know when you are safe to have unprotected intercourse. By following your own natural body rhythms
you can create a safe and reliable means of controlling
your fertility.

Why Use Natural Family Planning?

An ever increasing number of women and men are
becoming dissatisfied with their method of birth control and the choices available to them. Many are frightened about the potentially harmful effects of these
methods on the body. Some are concerned for moral
reasons. And some people are just interested in doing
things, including birth control, in a natural way.

Natural Family Planning is very simple from a scientific point of view, but so are many other things like
good diet, exercise and treating yourself well. Taking
the birth control pill fools your body by providing it
with artificial chemicals that make your body think
that it is going through the normal sexual cycle when
it really isn't. For many women this concept is offensive. The IUD presumably works to prevent the fertilized egg from implanting in the uterus. Thus, it is
very possible that each month a small but viable fetal
form is aborted due to the presence of the IUD. To
some this is offensive. And to a growing number of
women, any chemical or device from the outside placed
into the body seems wrong. For these people Natural
Family Planning is a way to return to a natural kind of
birth control without sacrificing much in the way of
safety (from unplanned pregnancy).

And finally, for those people who oppose any form
of artificial contraception (most notably the Roman
Catholic Church), this method is a perfect way to
control family size naturally. In our area many members of the Roman Catholic Church have supported
Natural Family Planning as a great advance over Calendar Rhythm. For these people and for the Catholic
doctors and scientists who have been in the forefront

of investigation into Natural Family Planning, this new contraception program represents the logical synthesis of science and ethics.

Who Can Use This New Birth Control Program?

Any woman who is willing to follow her natural body rhythms can use this new birth control program. It really doesn't matter how short, long or regular your cycles are. What is important is that you must be willing to follow these natural body rhythms each day, and to follow the rules of the program.

If you are dissatisfied with your current method of birth control we hope that Natural Family Planning will be a viable and emotionally satisfying method for you. This is especially true for women who have been on the pill or IUD and have worried about the medical side effects or had personal discomforts from them. Too often contraception has been at the expense of women. As every doctor knows, all the available methods of birth control carry some medical risks with their use. As one gynecologist put it, "Any time that you alter nature you pay a price. The price may be small or large." For some women the use of contraception has caused many serious medical problems. For others it has been only a problem of minor physical discomforts or fear of potential future dangers. We feel that the most important positive aspect of Natural Family Planning is that it does not invade the body with potentially harmful chemicals or devices, and therefore does not alter the natural functioning of the female body.

However, we also know that pregnancy carries with it a medical risk. Clearly the risk is necessary when women and men want to have children. However, the medical and emotional risks of an unplanned and unwanted pregnancy are not justifiable when effective methods of birth control are readily available. We want people to use Natural Family Planning in the most responsible and reliable way, or not to use it at all. For people who feel unable to follow their cycle on a regular basis and abstain from unprotected sexual intercourse when they are not safe, Natural Family Planning is not advised.

In the overall sense, we believe that Natural Family Planning can provide a new birth control alternative for people who have been dissatisfied with their current method(s) of contraception. We feel that it is medically safe and, if used properly, a highly effective means of controlling births. Our personal experience, and the experience of scientists and doctors in many parts of the world points to this in an overwhelming way.

Natural Family Planning and Calendar Rhythm

This new birth control method should not be confused with Calendar Rhythm, a method often associated with the Roman Catholic Church. Calendar Rhythm attempts to predict fertility by applying general rules to all women. Thus, a woman using Calendar Rhythm looks to a calendar to know when she is safe to have intercourse. If she uses the Ogino-Knaus method (discussed in Chapter Nine) she subtracts a fixed number of days from her longest and shortest cycles to find her safe time. Then she looks to the calendar to see when these safe days fall in the month. The Ogino-Knaus formula will probably work for most women for most of their cycles. However, since it represents the "average" woman, any woman who is not "average" for that month is very likely to become pregnant.

In contrast, Natural Family Planning allows you to follow your own individual and unique cycle. Since cycles vary among women and within the reproductive life of any individual woman, general rules of fertility are bound to have a relatively high rate of failure (unwanted pregnancy). No calendar can predict 100% of the time when you are safe or unsafe, and Calendar Rhythm has traditionally had a very high rate of failure (up to 60%) because of this. Natural Family Planning allows you to follow each cycle individually with no past or future events for comparison.

Thus, Natural Family Planning personalizes the concept of Calendar Rhythm. Each month you will be following your own cycle. You will be watching for your own changes, and can use these changes to determine when to have unprotected sex. If you follow a strict regime there is very little risk of having an unwanted pregnancy.

Natural Family Planning is the only method acceptable to the Roman Catholic Church, because it does not involve any artificial means of birth control. In fact, much of the pioneering work in this area has been accomplished by Catholic scientists and doctors who have been interested in finding a natural way of accurately knowing when a woman is safe. Thus, Natural Family Planning is not a break with the Church, but a great improvement over the Calendar Rhythm often taught as Church doctrine. We hope that the interest and influence of the Church in this area will continue to promote research into natural ways of following the female fertility cycle.

Contraceptive Overkill

While many people know that a woman is fertile sometime during the middle of her monthly cycle, few know that a woman ovulates only once each month, and that the egg she produces lives for only one to one-and-a-half days.

Most of the currently available methods of birth control are meant to be used every day of a woman's sexual life. This is a bizarre kind of "overkill" given the fact that a woman is able to conceive for only a fraction of the entire cycle. This new birth control program is based on the scientific notion that one can delineate the days of the month when a woman is fertile, and restrict the use of contraception (or abstinence) to those days.

The success of Natural Family Planning is based on

this natural cycle of infertile and fertile periods. We need only find more and better tests (and these tests must be inexpensive, simple and easy to perform) that women and men can employ to make Natural Family Planning a better and better means of birth control. It seems as if most doctors and researchers have considered overkill to be the only possible solution to the problem of contraception.

A Woman's Self-Awareness

Although the purpose of this new birth control program is to let you know when you can and cannot have unprotected sexual intercourse, an important secondary role is body self-awareness. The growth of feminism has had a profound effect in the area of women's health. Perhaps the most profound effect is the interest women have taken in their bodies and how they function. The Women's Self-Help Movement has done much to encourage women to know themselves better and be more prepared to defend their own best interest when seeking professional medical advice.

Natural Family Planning gives women an exciting way of following their sexual cycles. It is fascinating and gratifying to follow the regularity and individuality of your own cycle. Many women who have always thought of their cycle as erratic or irregular are surprised to find that they have an intrinsic regularity that they never knew existed. Chris has kept her own records of mood and energy level changes throughout her cycle. She has noted fluctuations, but of much more positive and dynamic nature than the traditional "premenstrual vapors" label put on any woman with a complaint or negative emotion. We feel that following the menstrual cycle is an exciting way of increasing your self-awareness that is an inevitable outgrowth of using this new program.

Family Planning for Men and Women Together

The burden of contraceptive risks and unwanted pregnancy has generally rested on women, and it is an old source of tension between couples. It is hard not to feel oppressed when the satisfaction of both people's sexual needs is dependent upon one person (the woman) taking a precaution that is often inconvenient, sometimes risky, and sometimes dangerous to her health.

Natural Family Planning is a method of contraception in which men and women share equally. Studies show that couples who have good communication in their relationship are much less likely to have an accidental pregnancy, and are much more likely to feel satisfied using the method. We do not believe that you have to be a couple to use Natural Family Planning successfully, but the ability to communicate with your partner is very likely to be the foundation for the success of this method of birth control. One couple put it very beautifully when they said, "We have three C's in our relationship, commitment, communication and consideration," and that Natural Family Planning had helped them develop this feeling. We believe that this new contraception program is a commitment to share the burden of birth control more equally between women and men in order to minimize the medical and psychological risks that have burdened women for so many years.

How We Became Interested

Chris knew about the temperature method from nursing school. She had been taught that women could take their temperature and follow their cycles in order to maximize the chance of conceiving by having intercourse at the right time. It was only after many years of using the diaphragm and disliking it that she began to think about using the temperature method as a way to follow her cycle to avoid conception.

Hank had hardly thought about an alternative to the diaphragm. He knew that Chris was opposed to an IUD, and we both had felt that the pill was potentially very dangerous. Moreover, Chris had tried taking the pill and had had many annoying side effects from it. So, when she suggested that she might start taking her temperature so that she could eventually reduce the number of days when she used a diaphragm, he was enthusiastic about the idea.

Chris took her temperature for six months before really using it as a method of birth control. Neither one of us really knew much about the science behind the temperature method and we were reluctant to dive right into it as a method of preventing conception. However, we began to "chip away" at the safe days of the cycle by having intercourse for a few days right after Chris's period ended. This was a bad idea, and we were very fortunate that Chris didn't have an unplanned pregnancy.

Our interest in the method grew as we began to follow the temperature chart. Hank attended a gynecology lecture where the doctor rated the temperature method (when used in the most careful and strict way) with the most highly effective methods, the pill and IUD. This convinced Hank that Natural Family Planning was actually good science. Then both of us began to read the scientific and medical literature on the subject and to expand our knowledge and interest.

By this time Chris was attending a Natural Family Planning course taught by a gynecologist and a woman who had been using it for a number of years. She brought many friends to these classes and was stimulated by their interest as well. Since many of her friends also wanted to find an alternative method of birth control, this program seemed to hold much promise.

Natural Family Planning has worked well for both of us. We use it ourselves and feel very good about it. Most of the time we don't have to use the diaphragm any more and feel happy to be done with it. We had always felt that it was inconvenient, unspontaneous and very messy. Now we only use it if we want to have intercourse on the unsafe days. Much of the unsafe time we make love without having intercourse. When one or the other of us has felt negative about the abstinence time we have tried to deal with it openly. We both feel that using Natural Family Planning is an investment in good health, sensible family planning and a positive future.

Beginning to Use this Book

If you are a person who likes to dive into the "how to" of things, you should go right on to Chapter Two and begin to learn how you can start following your cycle. If you are a person who gravitates towards personal stories, try starting with the interviews at the end of the book. These stories are told by people who use Natural Family Planning as their method of birth control. From their experiences you will begin to understand what his program means in terms of your life, your family and your health. In either case, we hope that you begin to delve into this new birth control program to see if it can provide you with a new way of relating to your body, fertility and sexuality.

CHAPTER TWO

How to Take and Chart Your Temperature

Developing a daily routine of taking your temperature is the first step of the New Birth Control Program. You will need to get in the habit of taking your awakening temperature every morning, except when you are having your period. By recording this morning basal temperature (called BBT), you can chart the biothermic changes taking place during your cycle. At first the routine might seem strange—doing something before you get out of bed in the morning—but soon you will find it no more difficult than taking a pill, remembering your house keys or brushing your teeth.

What Is Your Basal Body Temperature?

Your basal body temperature is the temperature of your body at rest. For some women this temperature can be obtained after six hours of rest, for others it might be shorter or longer. Since it is an "at rest" temperature, the BBT must be taken before any activity. This includes first thing trips to the bathroom, a cup of coffee or walking to the front door for the morning paper. Women with small children who use the program say they work out an arrangement with their partner so that he gets up initially with the child if it is early morning (time to take the temperature). That five-minute interval is one of his contributions to the working of the program.

For all women, the thing to remember is that to be most accurate:

> *Taking your BBT should be*
> *the first thing you do upon awakening.*

The BBT can be taken orally (by mouth) without any significant problems in accuracy and reliability. Some women have been concerned that breathing through the mouth (rather than through the nose) at night might make the temperature inaccurate. This does not seem to be the case in our experience. If you are a "mouth breather," you tend to sleep that way night after night, and the pattern is consistent for you. However, when you take your temperature, you should remember to place the thermometer well under your tongue and to keep your lips closed.

What Kind of Equipment Do You Need?

You will need a basal body thermometer to get good temperature readings. The basal body thermometer is a blown-up version of the usual household thermometer with the tenths of degree easily visible. The numbers go from 96.0 to 100.0 Fahrenheit (F). If you look at the basal body thermometer carefully you will note that the tenth of degree markings are larger than on a regular household thermometer, making it more accurate. This is important for the program user, since we are concerned with subtle changes that sometimes amount to only five or six tenths of a degree.

Basal body thermometers can be purchased at almost any drugstore. They range in price from $3.99 for a stripped-down model (less vivid markings, plastic case, no graph paper) to about $6 for a deluxe model with an insulated carrying case and a three-month's supply of chart paper. All the thermometers work pretty much the same, so the less expensive ones are better, given the breakage factor. If you travel a lot the insulated carrying case with a spring is handy. The preprinted graphs are useful, especially when you are first starting the program, but you can easily make your own on any piece of graph paper.

Taking Your Temperature

Taking, reading and recording your temperature is not difficult. The main trick is to be consistent in taking your temperature every day, without fail, and to remember to record it on your graph.

First, make sure that the thermometer has been shaken down completely. This is accomplished by holding the stem end (opposite from the bulb end) which you put in your mouth, firmly and shaking it in a "flick of the wrist" (staccato) motion. Caution should be taken to shake down your thermometer the night before so that it is ready for use in the morning. Don't be concerned that shaking the thermometer down in the morning will change your basal body temperature. The energy involved in shaking it down is negligible. What is important is that you don't wind up breaking it in a groggy morning shakedown. It is annoying, to say the least, to break your thermometer in the morning and miss your daily reading.

Second, place the thermometer in your mouth, with the bulb end under your tongue. Close your lips, not your teeth, and wait about five minutes before reading the temperature. Some women time by the clock, some by the length of one song on the clock radio. You'll find that it's nice to have a reason not to leap out of bed with the alarm.

Once the five minutes has passed, simply place the thermometer back in its holder to be read later. The thermometer will stay at the temperature you've taken until you shake it down, even if you let it sit for the day before making your recording.

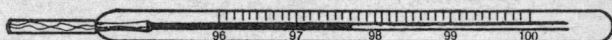

Figure 2 A basal body thermometer showing a temperature of 97.7F.

Reading the Thermometer

When you are ready to read the thermometer, simply hold it at eye level and slowly rotate the stem until the silver bar of mercury becomes visible. Looking from left to right, the number where the bar of mercury ends is your temperature.

In Figure 2, the bar of mercury is between the numbers 97 and 98. Remember that the lines between the numbers represent tenths of a degree and the numbers are whole degrees. So, counting from left to right, the bar falls seven line markings, or seven tenths of a degree over the 97. Therefore the reading is 97 plus seven tenths, or 97.7F.

If you have trouble reading your own thermometer at home it is probably because you have difficulty seeing the bar of mercury. Try rotating the thermometer in your fingers while looking carefully for the silver bar. Don't be discouraged if it takes a while to get used to—you'll catch on. Many doctors say that this program is not practical because some women can't take temperatures accurately and read them properly. However, these same women read their children's temperatures to pediatricians all the time. The most important thing is to keep doing it until taking and reading your temperature is second nature.

Recording Your Temperature

A graph is a scientific and mathematical way of making a series of observations. Making a graph from your daily basal body temperature readings is the first step in observing your menstrual cycle go through its changes in a way that makes sense. You will see your own

temperature pattern change with the dynamic alterations in your fertility.

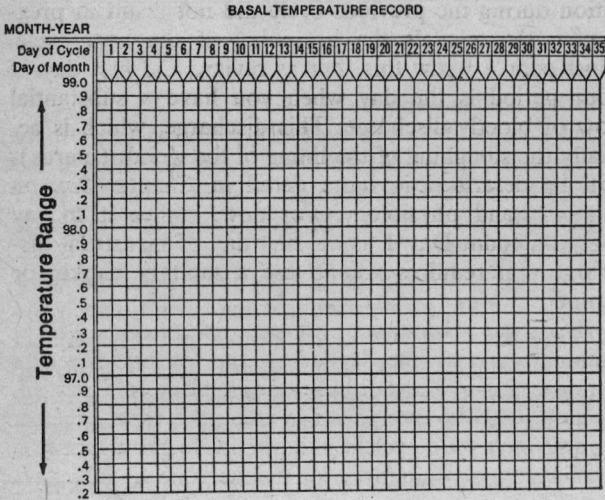

BASAL TEMPERATURE RECORD

MONTH-YEAR

Figure 3 A blank basal body temperature graph, with the degrees of
temperature range running from top to bottom and the days of the
cycle from left to right.

To record your temperatures you will need some kind
of graph paper and a pen or pencil. As seen in Figure
3, the graph is divided horizontally (across) into temperatures, and vertically (up and down) into days.
In marking the days across the top, notice that there
are two sets of numbers. The top numbers indicate the
days of the cycle. The numbers underneath represent
the calendar dates. It is important to have both sets of
days correctly in mind, so that if you, for example,
ovulate on day 14 of your cycle, you can correlate it
with a specific date, like March 9th.

The word "cycle" implies the circular rhythm of a
woman's fertility. The end of one cycle is, at the same
time, the beginning of the next. It is not linear, as the

graph might suggest, but a continuous repeating circle of events. *The first day of your period is called Day 1 of the cycle.* Thus, your period, which signals that ovulation during the previous cycle did not result in pregnancy, also signals the beginning of the next cycle. Most people know this, but as review, the first day of your period is the day when you have a substantial flow of bloody discharge. This discharge, which is actually the sloughing of the lining of the womb (uterus), will be described in more detail in Chapter Six, on anatomy and physiology. For now, suffice it to say that you count Day 1 as the first day of menstrual discharge that requires you to use a sanitary napkin or tampon.

If you are making your own charts, mark a sheet of graph paper with the days along the top and the temperatures along the side, just as it is done in Figure 3. Be sure to allow enough space along the "day" line for an unusually long cycle. Similarly, leave extra space on the line for temperatures for a fever due to infection. In general, the bigger your graph, the easier it is to see the changes. Allow plenty of space both in the days and the degrees to see the picture clearly.

Now look at Figure 4. This represents a woman's temperature for the first day after her period ended. As you see, Days 1 through 5 have been x'ed off. The first temperature recording is on Day 6 since it is not necessary to take your temperature during your period. Her temperature on Day 6 was 97.2F. She placed a dot where the Day 6 line met the 97.2 line. Notice that this also corresponds to the date May 12th.

You Can't Use the Pill!

Probably the hardest part about trying the New Birth Control Program is that you have to make a commitment to it before you can really use it. We advise that you follow your temperatures for a full six months (or six menstrual cycles) before you try to use it as a method of contraception. Moreover, you cannot take

BASAL TEMPERATURE RECORD

MONTH-YEAR *May / June 1975*

Day of Cycle	1	2	3	4	5	6	7	8	9	10	11	12	13	14	15	16	17	18	19	20	21	22	23	24	25	26	27	28	29	30	31	32	33	34	35
Day of Month	7	8	9	10	11	12	13	14	15	16	17	18	19	20	21	22	23	24	25	26	27	28	29	30	31	1	2	3	4	5	6	7	8	9	10

Period ✕✕✕✕✕

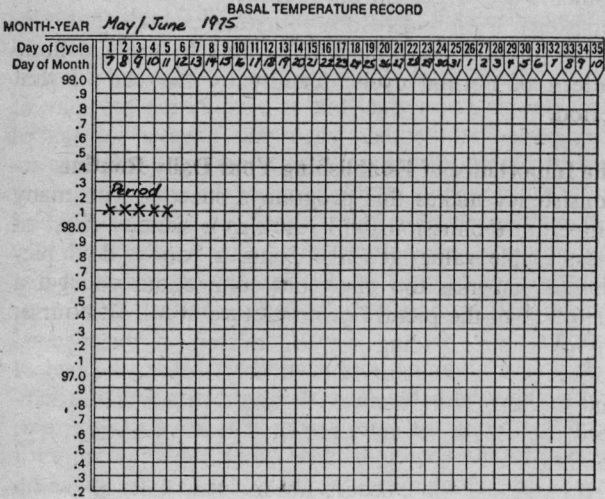

Figure 4 A graph showing a woman's temperature for the first day after her period has ended.

the birth control pill and have reliable temperature graphs. The pill is composed of hormones that control the basal body temperature, and when you take the pill it changes your natural biothermia.

You can, however, start taking and following your temperatures if you have an IUD, diaphragm or use condoms and contraceptive foams. As long as you are not taking the birth control pill or any other hormones, your temperature graph will accurately reflect your changing hormone levels. (The scientific basis for how hormones affect your temperature is explained in Chapter Six.) The pill will alter your natural basal body temperature, rendering your graphs inaccurate.

You shouldn't worry if your charts are a little confusing for the first few months after you stop taking the pill. The effects of the pill on your system do not stop the day you stop taking the pill. In fact, for many women, they linger on for months. Be patient and be persistent. Take and record your temperature faithfully for six months and you will be able to see a definite pattern of normal cyclic fertility by the end of that period.

The Importance of Establishing Your Daily Routine
Consistency makes this program a success. Too many temperature omissions will result in a sketchy chart of questionable value. It's like doing a "dot-to-dot" picture. If you miss too many dot connections you get a distortion of the picture or no picture at all. Of course, an occasional reading may be missed. If this occurs, note it on the chart under that date. Just make a note that the temperature wasn't taken, and continue to record the rest of the days for that month in the proper column.

If your omission occurs around the time of ovulation, you may lose a safe day. Don't try to fill in temperatures just because you think you know where they are, or what they should have been. Even if your chart this month looks a lot like last month's you shouldn't try to reuse last month's temperatures to fill in the gaps for this cycle. You may lose a safe day or two, but you insure the program's reliability.

Remember, the effectiveness of this method depends on you and your sexual partner. If you follow your body you won't go wrong. This means being aware each day, just as if you had to take a pill, insert a diaphragm or use a condom. The rules of the New Birth Control Program are simple and straightforward, but they are rather inflexible. Cheating on these rules can *definitely* result in an unplanned pregnancy.

Review
1. Your basal body or "at rest" temperature fluctuates during the month and these fluctuations are an indication of when you can and cannot get pregnant.

2. Your basal body temperature (BBT), taken daily with an oral thermometer, must be taken first thing upon awakening.

3. The first day of your period is considered the first day of your cycle.

4. BBT is recorded on a special graph. A dot is made where the line of the temperature crosses the line of the day on which this temperature was taken.

5. Many temperature omissions or use of oral contraceptives will result in an inaccurate graph that only sketchily, if at all, reflects fertility.

6. Trying to interpret an incomplete graph can result in an unplanned pregnancy.

7. It is necessary to make recording of six cycles of BBT patterns before beginning to use this program for contraception.

CHAPTER THREE

Reading Your Temperature Graphs: When It Is Safe to Resume Intercourse in the Cycle

The same hormones that make you fertile or infertile also change your temperature. Since the beginning of the twentieth century scientists have known that every woman's cycle is divided into times when she is fertile and can get pregnant and times when she is not fertile and cannot get pregnant. However, devising simple methods to tell you when you are infertile and therefore safe to have intercourse, has been the stumbling block to using this knowledge as a means of birth control.

Your temperature offers a way to use this knowledge, for it reflects the changes in your fertility.

IMPORTANT! *The temperature graph can only tell you when it is safe to have sexual intercourse AFTER you have ovulated.* It does not tell you about the time before ovulation. This part of the cycle is explained in Chapter Four, on the Mucus Method, and in the section on menstruation as a safe period.

How Does the Graph Tell You When You Are Safe?
Look at the graph in Figure 5. It illustrates a 28 day

cycle. The first temperature recorded is 97.9F. After
Day 6, the temperature sort of jags up and down, but
basically stays between 97.6 and 97.9 until Day 15.
From Day 15 onward, the temperature takes a definitive rise to around 98.3 and stays in this higher range
until the next period begins.

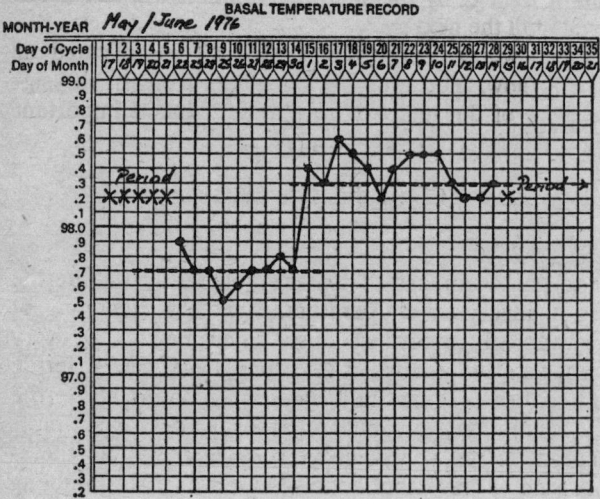

Figure 5 A twenty-eight day cycle. The lower dotted line represents
the preovulatory baseline before the temperature rise on day
fifteen. The higher dotted line represents the post-ovulatory baseline.

*The temperature rise that occurred on Day 15 was
due to changes in sex hormones that determine fertility. It indicates that ovulation has occurred for
the cycle.*
Once you know that you have ovulated, you can figure
when it is safe to start having intercourse again.

The temperature rise shown in Figure 5 represents a definitive rise in the basal body temperature. This thermic shift, as it is called, is the important information that tells you when you can and cannot get pregnant. After your temperature goes up and stays up, you are on the infertile period of your cycle. You cannot get pregnant during the infertile period because your body is producing hormones that are unfavorable to fertilization of the egg by the sperm. Ovulation will not occur again until the next cycle.

Don't worry if this all seems a bit complicated or unclear now. You are only beginning to learn the significance of the temperature graph. What is important to realize is that the temperature graph can tell you when you have ovulated, i.e. when your fertile time has passed, and it is safe to have intercourse.

The Biphasic Curve

A Biphasic curve is one in which there are two levels or distinct areas. If you look at Figure 5, you will see that from menses (period to Day 14, the temperature is definitely lower than from Day 15 until the next period, which starts on Day 29. This early, lower temperature is your preovulatory (before ovulation) temperature. The temperature after is a higher, postovulatory (after ovulation) temperature.

A good way to see the two levels of the biphasic curve is to get an "eyeball average" of the pre- and postovulatory temperatures with a pencil or ruler. Look again at Figure 5. Notice the two horizontal lines. The lower line is drawn across the average temperature or the *preovulatory baseline* of those first nine recorded temperatures. The higher line is the average point of the temperatures between Day 15 and Day 28. This is the *postovulatory baseline*.

Pre- and postovulatory baselines give your cycle this biphasic temperature graph.

What Does the Rise Mean?

The temperature shift represents the change your body goes through when it stops producing lots of estrogen and starts producing progesterone. These two hormones change your body from an environment in which sperm can penetrate the egg, producing a pregnancy, to one in which sperm cannot live and move. (A more in-depth discussion of these two hormones may be found in Chapter Six.)

For now, be aware that the temperature change tells you that you have already ovulated for that cycle and that you are producing hormones that make it unfavorable for the sperm to reach and penetrate the egg (even if there were one). Thus, the elevated part of your temperature cycle is the time when unprotected intercourse is safe and a pregnancy will not occur.

When Are You Safe in the Biphasic Curve?

After your temperature has risen from the pre-ovulatory baseline six tenths of a degree for three successive days, you are safe to have unprotected intercourse.

The three-day wait serves two purposes:

First, it allows for the lifespan of the egg, believed to be from 12 to 36 hours.

Second, it allows for certainty of a definitive temperature rise. After three days, the user can be sure that it is truly the hormonal change causing the shift rather than some other factor, like fever, a restless night, etc.

Look back to Figure 5 and notice that the temperature rise on Day 15 is followed by a slight dip on Day 16. This lower temperature might be due to some basal body variation, but it still remains above the average preovulatory baseline. Furthermore, on Days 17 and 18, the temperature is up again to the six tenths degree rise range. Clearly the hormonal shift has occurred and conception (and pregnancy) can no longer occur. For this woman, intercourse was safe on Day 18, and from then on until her next period.

BASAL TEMPERATURE RECORD

MONTH-YEAR *February / March 1975*

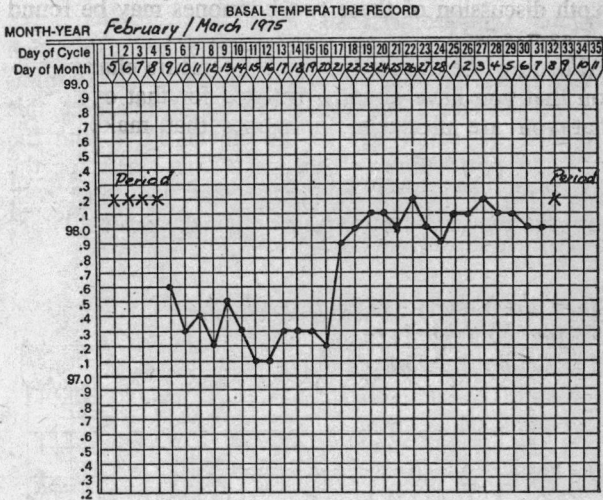

Figure 6 A graph showing a sustained rise of six tenths of a degree for three days. On day nineteen intercourse without protection will be safe.

In Figure 6, the temperature shift occurs somewhat later in the month. Try to visualize that the preovulatory temperature is around 97.2F until Day 17. On Day 17, the temperature goes up to 97.9 and stays up on Day 18 also. Although the temperature varies a bit, it basically remains elevated. Therefore, on Day 19, when the temperature has been up three days, inter-

course without protection will be safe. Remember that
the rule is that you are safe after

> *a sustained rise of six tenths of a degree*
> *for three days.*

This sustained rise is our rule of thumb for finding the
postovulatory safe time for unprotected intercourse.

Gradual Temperature Rise

Now, look at Figure 7. This shows a cycle in which
the temperature went up slowly, cutting down the number of safe days somewhat. You still interpret this
graph in the same way as the others. First, find the
pre- and postovulatory baselines. Then, look for the
rise. And, of course, remember that you must wait
until the temperature range is within the postovulatory

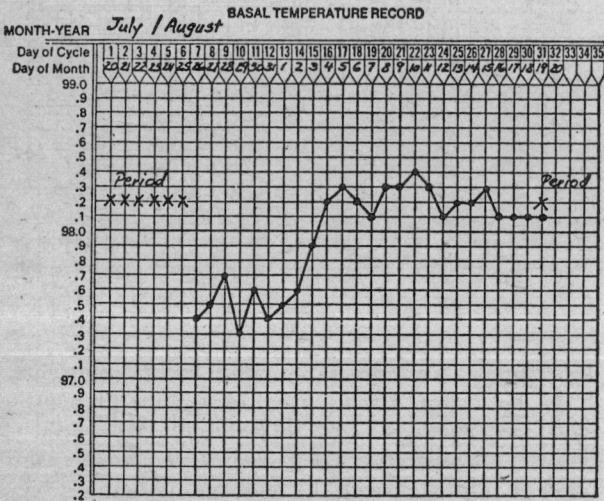

Figure 7 In this cycle the temperature goes up slowly.

baseline range for three days before you can determine that you are no longer fertile.

In this graph, (Figure 7), the temperature starts to rise on Day 15, but only a 0.3 degree rise. On Day 16, though, it is up to 98.2F, which is a six tenths degree difference from the preovulatory baseline. Although Day 15 is indeed part of the postovulatory rise, you cannot count it as Day 1 when calculating when you are safe. Day 16 is counted as the first day of the rise, so intercourse is safe in this instance on Day 18.

The Fall Before the Rise

At the time of ovulation, there is a small dip in the body's temperature. If you ovulate in the morning, just prior to taking your BBT, your graph will show this

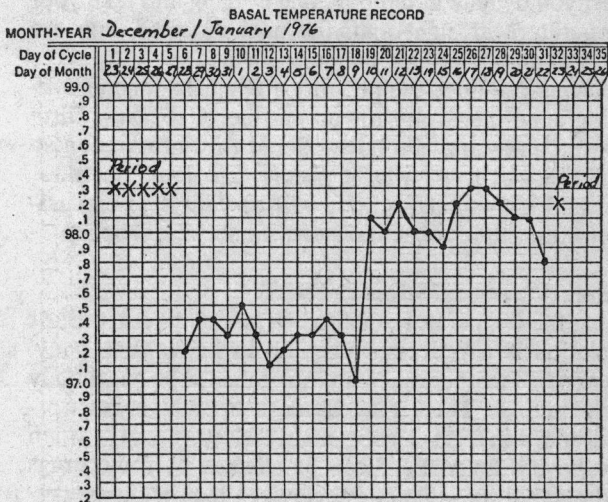

Figure 8 In this graph there is a slight drop in temperature on day eighteen, just before the post-ovulatory rise.

slight dip of several tenths of a degree. The next BBT you take will show the characteristic rise and should stay up for the rest of the cycle. This dip at the time of ovulation is normal.

Look at Figure 8. In this graph you can see that on Day 18 there is a slight drop in temperature, followed on Day 19 by the familiar postovulatory rise. You should note that the temperature after this dip represents Day 1 of the sustained rise. Therefore, intercourse would be safe on Day 21.

If your graphs do not always (or seldom) show this dip in temperature you should not be concerned, since finding the dip in temperature associated with ovulation depends on lucky timing. Chris has noted an ovulatory dip only infrequently. If you ovulate at six a.m. and take your temperature at 8 a.m. that same day, you are likely to notice this slight temperature drop. If, however, you ovulate at ten p.m. one evening and take your temperature at eight a.m. the next morning, you are likely to miss this slight temperature dip.

Seeing the dip in temperature around the time of ovulation is not necessary for proper use of the New Birth Control Program. We have offered this information so that you will know why it occurs if it does. For now, just add it to what we hope will be your ever-expanding awareness of ways to observe your cyclic changes.

Fevers, Illness and Stress and BBT

Using the temperature method to pinpoint your time of ovulation is a process of getting to know your body. Clearly, all temperatures are not going to be basal body temperatures. There may be days when you are worried and don't get a good night's sleep, or days when you have a fever. BBT can be affected by some drugs and alcohol as well. These elevated temperatures cannot tell you anything about your ovulation point. You should chart them on the graph, but note the circumstances under which they were taken.

MONTH-YEAR *September*   BASAL TEMPERATURE RECORD

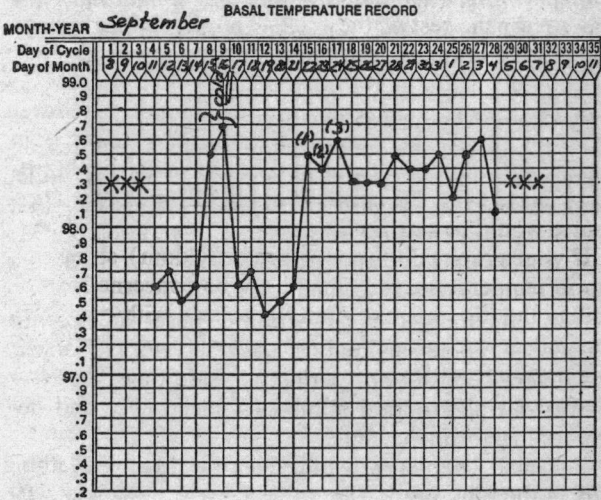

Figure 9 This graph shows a temperature variation caused by an arti-fact, in this case: a cold.

Figure 9 shows how we suggest using your graph when there is a question of the reliability of a given day's BBT. Merely mark on the graph that you think you had a fever, bad night's sleep, stayed up late partying, or whatever, next to the temperature for that morning. When you interpret your graph for that cycle, be suspicious about these temperatures that you have noted, particularly if they don't follow the pattern. It is *always better* to wait an extra day or two before having unprotected intercourse than to risk an unplanned pregnancy.

As you begin to know your body's baseline temperatures, these inappropriate readings (called *artifacts*) will become more apparent. Just remember that they should be disregarded when looking for your post-ovulatory rise. Thus, *drugs, alcohol, illness and stress may result in inappropriate temperatures and they should not be used when looking for your postovulatory safe period.*

A System of Checks and Balances

As you can see, the temperature method requires an average abstinence period of about half of the cycle. Looking back to Figure 6, the graph indicates that unprotected intercourse is safe from Day 19 to Day 31. This is 13 safe days and 18 unsafe days in a 31 day cycle. This is a little less than half safe days.

By combining the temperature observation with knowledge about anatomical and secretory changes, and determining if your period is a safe time, the New Birth Control Program minimizes uncertainty and decreases the abstinence time.

The next chapter will introduce the Mucus Method part of the program.

Review

1. Your normal ovulating body temperature will give a biphasic curve. This curve has two phases or areas: a preovulatory, lower temperature baseline and a postovulatory, higher temperature baseline.

2. After your temperature has risen six tenths of a degree for three consecutive days, you are no longer fertile for the rest of that cycle.

3. The basal body "at rest" temperature may be altered by some drugs, alcohol, illness, a restless night or other stress factors.

4. Beware of temperatures that seem to contradict your normal pattern. If you are uncertain about a temperature for any reason, mark it on the graph. If this questionable temperature occurs around the time of ovulation, wait an extra day(s) to be sure before having unprotected intercourse.

5. The temperature method of the program tells you when you can start having intercourse again AFTER OVULATION TAKES PLACE. It cannot predict ovulation, it can only determine that it has taken place.

CHAPTER FOUR

Preovulation: The Mucus Method

The BBT can only tell you when ovulation has *occurred,* and when you are safe to have unprotected intercourse in the latter part of your cycle. You can also monitor the changes in your menstrual cycle by observing the quality and quantity of your vaginal secretions. Most of us are unaware that the discharge from the vagina varies with the time of the month. Indeed, many women do not realize that this discharge is a normal part of their fertility cycle. These "vaginal" secretions actually come from the glands in the cervix (lower part of the uterus or womb). The amount of the secretion and, more importantly, the chemical composition of this secretion (called *mucus*), is controlled by the female hormones. These hormones, in turn, fluctuate with the cycle.

One type of mucus is hospitable, encouraging to the life of sperm. This fertile mucus, at its peak around the time of ovulation, allows sperm to pass easily through it and make its way through the uterus and into the fallopian tubes where it can penetrate the egg. Look at Figure 10. The drawing at the left is a schematic representation of this fertile mucus. Spaces are large, and the configuration is channellike, allowing sperm to move easily about. Now, look at the drawing to the right. This represents mucus during the nonfertile periods. It appears as a tangled, tight mass and, as is shown, even the tiny sperm cell cannot penetrate it. If the sperm cell cannot penetrate this mucus at the opening of the uterus, it cannot swim to the fallopian tubes. Conception in the absence of the hospitable mucus, then, is not possible.

There are other variabilities of cervical mucus besides viscosity (thickness). Most of the time the vagina tends to be too acidic for sperm to live in. What many contraceptive jellies, creams and foams do is change the acidity and secretions of the vagina so conception is less likely to occur. Without the use of these synthetic chemicals, the cervical secretions become more basic

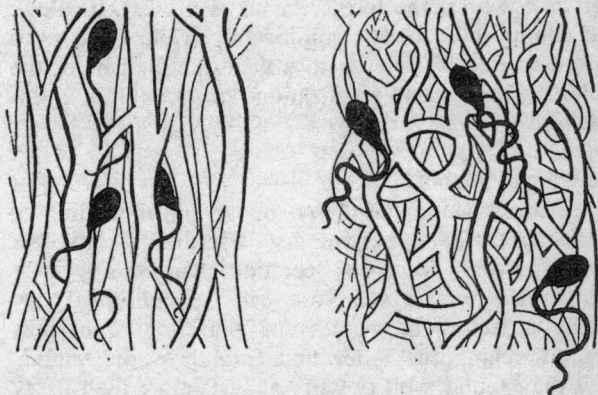

Figure 10 On the left, a sperm swimming through fertile mucus. On the right, the sperm is unable to penetrate the infertile mucus.

(or nonacid) as the ovulation time approaches. It is the function of the mucus to change the vagina from acidic to basic so the sperm can live. The mucus also gives the sperm nutrients to use in its travels.

*Sperm can live up to five days
in mucus that is hospitable.*

This is a very important fact to remember when calculating safe and unsafe times. If the mucus is hospitable, one could have intercourse five days before ovulation and still conceive!

To review, each time a man ejaculates, he releases a moderate amount of thickish milky secretion called semen. This semen, which is a nourishing environment for sperm, can hold up to 400,000,000 of these sperm cells. It takes several hours for the sperm that is deposited in a woman's vagina at the time of ejaculation to swim through the cervix and uterus and into the fallopian tubes. If the vaginal environment is hostile, the sperm are quickly immobilized and are thus unable to make the journey to the spot where the egg might be. If, however, the fertile mucus is present, it allows the sperm cells to live comfortably while they move toward the egg, and even to wait in the far part of the fallopian tube where fertilization occurs until an egg is released.

Looking at Mucus

The Mucus Method is based on an understanding of the changes that we have just described. It involves keeping a daily record of secretion changes. For some women the mucus symptom can be "observed" by noting a feeling of wetness or a feeling of dryness when touching the inner lips (labia) of the vagina. This may sound a bit obscure at first; more than likely you have never correlated these sensations with your fertility cycle. This "wetness" is not to be confused with the lubricant that appears in the vagina when you are sexually aroused. Rather it is a perceived wetness during a neutral part of your day.

Try it for awhile. Take a moment out during the day to be aware of this wetness or dryness: the presence or absence of cervical mucus. Some women we know say that they can tell if they are wet or dry "no hands" by just thinking of how they feel. Others say they first related the mucus to the change in the discharge that they noted on their underwear throughout the cycle.

Note your observations, perhaps on your temperature graph, and see if you can see a pattern in your mucus as it changes from wet to dry.

Many women find it helpful to actually look at the mucus. Whether you use this method will depend on your feelings about touching your genitals. If you want to observe the changes in this way, you can take a sample of mucus from the back of the vagina or from the cervix itself. This is accomplished by inserting your middle finger into the vagina until you feel the small "bump" that is your cervix. Don't be afraid to insert the finger in all the way. It can be quite far back in some women. How far back it is also varies according to where you are in your cycle (this will be discussed later in the chapter). Don't be afraid that you will hurt yourself. The cervix is not hard to locate with a little patience, and a mucus sample is not hard to obtain.

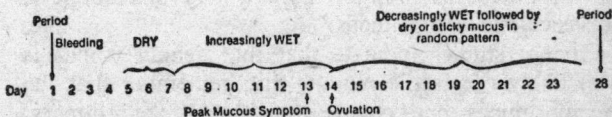

Figure 11 The mucus cycle.

What You Will See

Based on a cycle that starts with Day 1 as the first day of your period, the mucus cycle is roughly as follows (see Figure 11): Day 1 through Day 5 are bleeding from the menstrual period. Right after menses, secretions are greatly decreased (almost absent) and the vagina feels dry. It might feel a bit irritating to insert the last tampon. For some women, intercourse at this time may be difficult due to the dryness. This is a dryness separate from lubrication during sexual arousal. As you see in Figure 11, Days 6 and 7 are noted as "dry" on the chart.

Dry days mean the absence of fertile mucus.

Therefore, sexual intercourse during dry days would not result in conception. If the sperm could survive the acid vagina, it could not penetrate the tightly meshed mucus at the cervical opening.

These two, three or more postmenstrual dry days are followed by the expulsion of a mucus plug from the opening of the cervix. You may not notice this small, sticky plug, but you *will* notice the change in secretions following its expulsion. This new secretion, which makes the lips (labia) of the vagina feel wet, increases in its slipperiness and stretchability as you proceed towards ovulation (release of the egg).

Some women note that the first mucus after the dry days in whitish and sticky or "tacky." On the chart, this woman has noted such mucus on Days 8, 9 and 10. Now notice that starting with Day 11, she identifies the mucus as thinner, more watery and slippery. This is classic fertile mucus.

Current studies indicate that the creamy mucus is most likely not fertile mucus. But, remember that the creamy mucus can change quickly to the slippery, fertile type—and, anyway, "probably" doesn't sound too reassuring when we are talking about the possibility of an unplanned pregnancy. Our guideline is to

*stop unprotected intercourse after
the appearance of any mucus symptoms!*

For this woman, unprotected intercourse would end on Day 8.

On Day 13 the mucus is described as "egg white in appearance." Peak cervical mucus takes on the appearance of the white of an uncooked egg. It is clear, somewhat gelatinous and slippery. This mucus is also stretchy. If you place a small amount between your thumb and first finger, and slowly pull your fingers apart, the mucus will stretch—for some people up to 10 cm. (about 4 inches) in length. This mucus symptom, called spinnbarkeit, is present just prior to ovulation. It usually occurs the day before you will ovulate. On this chart, the woman has noted this peak mucus symptom on Day 13. On Days 14, 15 and 16 she notes a change in the secretion to less slippery, more creamy. This indicates a return to the dense, more acid, nonfertile mucus. She also notes some dry days again before her period starts.

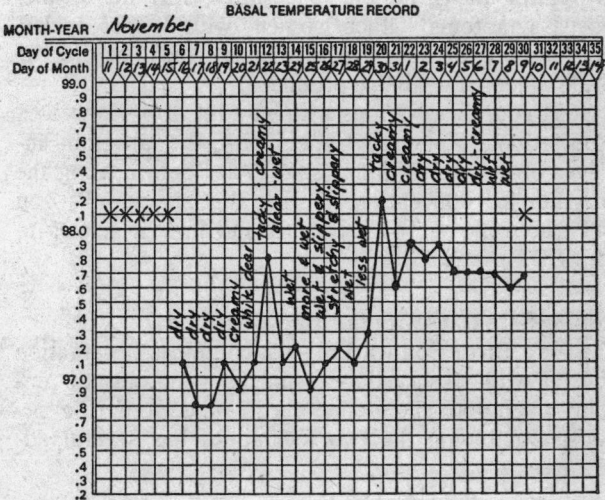

Figure 12 The mucus cycle shown on a temperature graph.

Looking at Mucus and Temperature Changes Together

Figure 12 shows the mucus symptom superimposed on the BBT record of this woman's same cycle. As you can see, the peak mucus symptom coincided exactly with the day before the temperature indicated that she ovulated. Note also that the postovulatory mucus changes vary from white to dry to wet to creamy. Mucus is variable AFTER ovulation, but this is not a problem, since the fertility period has already occurred for this cycle.

A Word About Each Woman's Uniqueness

As with the BBT your mucus pattern will follow a pattern that is unique to you. The outline above is just that; a sketch of what the pattern will be. You will fill in the sketch with your own individual fertility pattern. Some women with very short cycles have no dry days after menstruation, but start with the creamy mucus symptoms. Other women, with longer cycles, have 5 or 6 dry days after their periods, before the fertile mucus starts being produced.

Start your observations without a lot of preconceived expectations. Remember that using the program involves observing six months of cycles before using the program for conception. During this six months you will discover your own pattern and how it relates to your BBT graph.

Adding Safe Days with the Mucus Method

The New Birth Control Program combines observation of BBT with observation of mucus symptoms to pinpoint ovulation and define fertile and nonfertile periods. Combining the two techniques has several advantages:

First of all, mucus observation adds safe days to the cycle. As we have said, BBT observation cannot *predict* ovulation. With temperature observation alone, you would have to stop intercourse before or right after menstrual flow ceases. But, knowing that dry days are inhospitable to the life of sperm allows one or more postmenstrual days as safe days.

Secondly, the mucus method serves as a check on the BBT method, when BBT is raised due to infection or medication. It also is indispensable for use during menopause and lactation (breast-feeding), when temperatures can be erratic (see Chapter Five).

Thirdly, BBT can be used when vaginal infection makes mucus observation difficult.

Fourth, and most important, mucus observation with BBT observation provides a dynamic of checks and balances that can make you more secure while using the program. Clearly, a method that creates a constant fear of pregnancy is not acceptable. We believe that it is the combination of various ways of observing the fertility cycle that will make New Birth Control Program users feel secure.

Starting to Make Mucus Observations

Oral contraceptives change the vaginal secretions as well as altering the BBT. One cannot get a meaningful record of cervical secretion changes while taking oral contraceptives. Some women experience a lot of vaginal infections and break-through bleeding (bleeding between periods) with the IUD which can also make secretion observation difficult, though not impossible. And, unfortunately, contraceptive creams, jellies and foams add a synthetic secretion that can be confused with cervical mucus.

Some women say that, with practice, cervical mucus changes can be noted in spite of other secretions present, including semen. However, we recommend that initially you refrain from sexual intercourse during the preovulatory period for one or more cycles to get an idea of what you are looking for. After this trial period, try observing the mucus symptom after a substantial period of time following sexual intercourse. For example, if you have intercourse on Tuesday

night, wait until Wednesday evening to make your
mucus observation. By that time most of the semen
would have been discharged from your vagina and
mucus from the cervix will bè easier to see.

Get used to describing what the mucus looks like.
Note the color (whitish, clear, yellow, blood-tinged),
the amount (slight, moderate, profuse) the texture and
the appearance (thin, thick, slippery, stretchy, curdled,
jellylike). Try to compare today's mucus symptom with
yesterday's and note the changes. Some women experience light spot bleeding at midcycle around the time of
ovulation. This will, of course, affect the mucus symptom.

*Midcycle spotting cannot be absolutely
associated with the day of ovulation.*

We do not suggest using it to pinpoint ovulation, but it
can surely be used as another correlating symptom.

Other Noteworthy Changes that Reflect Your Fertility Cycle

Besides temperature and mucus changes, other mani-
festations of the cycle are known. The cervix, which is
the muscular extension of the uterus that projects to
the back of the vagina, actually changes position during
the cycle. After menses, the cervix is low in the vagina.
You will find it is easily touched if you put your finger
into your vagina a relatively short distance. This can
also make the insertion of last-day tampons feel irritating. The vagina seems to have less room than usual.
This sensation is due to the low position of the cervix.

The opening of the cervix, called the os, is closed
right after menses and the cervical tissue feels firm
(about the texture of the tip of your nose). As the
cycle moves into its preovulatory phase, the cervix is
pulled upward by a pair of ligaments that hold it in
place in the pelvis. This causes the cervix to be drawn
up and toward the back of the vagina. Now, if you
insert your finger, the cervix seems much further back,

even slightly out of reach. Cervical texture becomes softer (the consistency of your upper lip) and the os opens up again the breadth of a fingertip to make it easier for the sperm to gain entrance to the uterus (the degree to which the os opens often depends on whether or not you have ever had a baby: opened more if you have, less if you haven't).

If you are interested in following these changes, they add another dimension to the picture of how your body procedes through the fertility cycle. Cervical position changes are summarized in Figure 13 and in the interview with Dr. Furlong in Chapter Eleven.

Fertile	Not Fertile
High	Lower
Soft (like your lip)	Firm (like your nose)
Open (To a finger tip)	Closed
Wet	Dryer
Slippery	Not Slippery
Not Safe for Intercourse	Safe for Intercourse

Figure 13 A summary of cervical changes from fertility to infertility.

Ferning Patterns of Cervical Mucus

If you took a sample of your cervical mucus at the time of ovulation and looked at it under a microscope, you would see that it crystallizes in a pattern that remarkably resembles the ferns you might find during a walk in the woods. This ferning is another good measurement of your place in your cycle. If you ovulate on Day 14, for example, you would have little ferning until Day 7 or so. From that time on, the amount of crystallization and ferning would increase as you moved toward ovulation. It would peak at ovulation with the "forest fern" pattern. After ovulation, it decreases, losing the fern configuration.

The fern pattern is controlled by the same hormones that we have been discussing all along. As you proceed toward ovulation, you produce more nutritive mucus containing proteins, sugars and salts which nourish the sperm and change the acidity of the vagina. The more you have of this sugar and protein mucus, the more the chemical strands cross and link, producing the ferning pattern.

It is obvious that most of us don't have access to a microscope to observe ferning pattern. We mention it here to underline the fact that our bodies are rhythmical and predictable with changes that we can see in a variety of ways.

Mittelschmertz

Many women report a slight cramping feeling, low and on either side of the abdomen, around the middle of the cycle. This cramp, called mittelschmertz (German, for middle pain), results from the rupture of the egg out of the ovary (see Chapter Six for a detailed discussion of ovulation). Like the midcycle spot bleeding,

> *the presence of mittelschmertz does not necessarily pinpoint the day of ovulation!*

Studies have shown that some women experience this cramping several days before or after actual ovulation. Make note of mittelschmertz symptoms on your own chart and see how it relates to your ovulation day.

Menstruation as a Safe Period

We mentioned in Chapter One that for most women, the menstrual period is a safe time. Before continuing, we should say more about using the menstruation time for unprotected intercourse.

The question of whether or not to have intercourse during the period is an old and controversial one. Many women use menses as a time to engage in sexual intercourse without chemicals or devices. They reason that if ovulation is in the middle of the month, menstration is way to one side of the fertile period. They also figure that when the lining of the uterus is being shed and expelled, it would be hard for the sperm to reach the egg (swimming upstream and all), and hard for a fertilized egg to implant in the uterine wall.

This reasoning is certainly not illogical, but there remains a nagging doubt, accentuated by the occasional story we hear of the woman who swears that the only time she could have possibly conceived her last child was during her period.

What is menstruation? It is the shedding of the lining of the uterus because fertilization has not occurred. It is the result of a failed ovulation. We think of ovulation coming a certain time after our period, but, in reality, it is the other way around. Our period occurs a certain amount of time after ovulation, unless a fertilized egg implants in the uterus. In fact, for most women, menses regularly comes a certain number of days (around two weeks) after the day of ovulation. So when your period comes earlier than usual, it means you ovulated earlier than usual (for you.) Conversely, a later period would indicate that you ovulated later in that cycle.

What does this have to do with safety? Well, if your period comes about two weeks after you ovulate, your cycle length could tell you about when you tend to ovulate each cycle. Statistically, the day of ovulation falls on a bell curve. This means that the highest percentage of women will ovulate on Day 14. However, a substantial number will ovulate on each side of Day 14, on Days 12, 13, 15 or 16, for example. As we move out from the center, the number of women ovulating at statistically unusual times (unusual for the entire population, not unusual for you) decreases. Thus very few women ovulate on Day 22 or Day 8, BUT SOME WOMEN DO.

The late ovulation does not concern us when discussing menses safety, but early ovulation does. If you happen to be someone who ovulates on Day 7 or 8 or even 9 or 10, you could indeed conceive while having intercourse during your period, if the fertile mucus was present. Let's say you have a six day period and have intercourse on the last day. Menstrual blood is alkaline (basic) and so it is not hostile to sperm. But, since it is not particularly helpful either, the fertile mucus would have to be present to help the sperm reach an egg in the fallopian tube. Thus, if your body ovulates early, on Day 9, the fertile mucus could be present and conception could take place. Moreover, you would not know that the mucus is present, since the menstrual blood would cover it up. But it could be there, and the sperm deposited on Day 6 would live to Day 9 when ovulation would occur.

Deciding on Safety During Menses

There is a way to determine the likelihood of conceiving during your menstrual period. It is our method of estimating whether or not you are ovulating just after your period ends, and will give you an idea of whether the menstrual period is a safe time. It is only a guideline since the menstrual flow can obscure the presence of mucus, making conception possible. Use this formula to decide whether to have unprotected intercourse during menses, understanding that there is a potential risk of pregnancy.

Since menstruation results from the failure to conceive during the cycle, the time from ovulation to the next menstrual period is relatively fixed. To judge whether your period is safe look over your cycles for the past six months and note the longest number of days from your ovulation until the period. Also note the length of your shortest cycle. Subtract the longest interval from your ovulation until your period from the length of the shortest cycle, to determine the earliest day of ovulation. Then subtract another five days to allow for the life of sperm in favorable mucus. If this day falls at a time when you are having menstrual flow, you must be aware that your flow will cover the presence of fertile mucus. In this case conception is a possibility and unprotected intercourse is not safe.

Let's go through some examples that will help make this concept easier to understand. Let's say that during six months of observation your shortest cycle is 26 days, and your longest interval between ovulation and your next menstrual period is 15 days. Subtracting 26 minus 15, you get that your earliest day of ovulation is Day 11. Then subtracting five days for the life of sperm, you are safe up until Day 6. However, if you have an eight day period you could not tell whether or not you are having fertile mucus on Days 6, 7 and 8, and unprotected intercourse is not advisable. If, however, you have a five day period, you will be able to know if you are wet (fertile mucus present) or dry on Day 6, and can determine whether intercourse is safe. To review this example:

> Shortest cycle is 26 days by observation of *at least* 6 months
> Longest interval from ovulation to the next period is 15 days
> 25 - 15 = 11, earliest estimated day of ovulation
> 11 - 5 (Days when sperm can live in fertile mucus) = 6. Thus, Day 6 is the last safe day during the beginning of the cycle when intercourse is safe, if you cannot observe your mucus due to menstrual flow.

Let's say that in this example the woman abstains during Day 6, her period ends, and she is able to observe her mucus. If she observes that she is "dry" she is then able to resume having intercourse until she sees the onset of "wet days," or what we call the fertile mucus.

Here's another example. This woman's shortest cycle was 21 days, and her longest interval between ovulation and her next period was 14 days. Thus,

> Shortest cycle = 21 days
> Longest interval between ovulation and next period is 14 days
> 21 - 14 = 7, earliest likely day of ovulation
> 7 - 5 (Days when sperm can live in favorable mucus) = 2

In this example she is safe for the first day of her period, but should wait from Day 2 until her period ends before having unprotected intercourse. Once her period ends she can observe her mucus to see if the "wet" or favorable mucus is present. If she is dry she is safe to have intercourse.

For women with longer cycles this calculation emphasizes the safety of intercourse during the menstrual period. For example, let's look at a situation where the shortest cycle is 32 days and the longest interval between ovulation and the next menses is 15 days.

32 (shortest cycle - 15 (period of ovulation to next menses) = 17
17 (earliest day of ovulation) - 5 (life of sperm in mucus) = 12

This woman is safe from the onset of her period to Day 12. Thus if she has a five day period her entire menstrual period is very likely to be safe, and she will be able to check her mucus symptoms long before she is likely to ovulate.

This method of estimation is our method of evaluating the likelihood of ovulating or having fertile mucus present during your menstrual period. It is clearly not as safe as abstaining from unprotected intercourse during the period and waiting for the "dry" days. Thus, judgment about the possibility of getting pregnant during your period is very individual and based on your own menstrual pattern. Overall, it is safest not to attempt to predict the future ovulation on the basis of past ovulations. And, to be completely safe one would have to abstain from any intercourse during the menses until the cervical secretions can be seen without competition from the menstrual flow. It is worthwhile to evaluate your own menstrual cycles to realize that early ovulation makes intercourse during your period less likely to be safe, and that complete safety is not assured unless you can evaluate your mucus symptoms unencumbered by the menstrual flow. Statistically ovulation during menstruation is rare, but it does occur. We hope that the information contained in this section will help you make that judgment for yourself.

One More Caution

One more caution about intercourse during a period is necessary. As we have mentioned, some women experience a small amount of midcycle bleeding at the point of ovulation. If you are not in touch with the changes in your cycle, you might see this spotting as the first day of your period and have unprotected intercourse. You are very likely to become pregnant if you do have intercourse at this time. This may seem far-fetched, but we have been told by doctors that this miscalculation accounts for many of the "I got pregnant during my period" stories. This problem should be eliminated for women who carefully follow their cycles with basal body temperature graphing and mucus observations. In these cases, it should be obvious that this midcycle bleeding is occurring with ovulation, not menstruation.

A Summary of Various Symptoms

Take a minute to look at Figure 4-6. This chart summarizes the various aspects of cervical mucus and the position of the cervix throughout the fertility cycle. Refer back to this chart as you create your own graph of fertility observations.

Putting All of Your Observations Together

By now you may feel that you need a spiral notebook in diary form to record all the information about cycle changes. Although it may seem when you first read this that you will be using the greater part of your day thinking about fertility, this is not the case. "Observation" of some symptoms, like mucus and mittelschmertz, may involve no more than noting the cramping mentally and charting it later, or taking a moment out each day to look at the mucus or mentally noting whether the day is wet or dry for you.

There are a variety of ways of keeping track of fertility changes. Some women keep a sheet of paper with daily recordings of mucus, cervical changes and/or mood and energy changes. Temperature changes are graphed on a separate piece of paper. Chris prefers combining these observations by printing mucus and other changes on the BBT graph. At times when she has gotten into noting a lot of mood and energy changes she uses a separate sheet, but generally she tries to keep everything in one space so that she can see a whole picture of the cycle.

Experiment with different ways of recording and see what feels best. We encourage you to keep neat, orderly records. This is essential for preventing pregnancy. It also provides a clear record of your individual cycle that can be read at a later date, or shared with other women interested in this program.

Use All the Information You Can Get

Although there are different observations you can make, we suggest using BBT and mucus symptoms together as a basis for success and safety with the program. Beyond that, use all of the information you can get to help you understand the dynamic changes throughout your cycle.

Review

1. Changes occurring in the mucus found in the vagina can tell you when you can and when you cannot get pregnant.

2. Infertile mucus is too dense and too acid for sperm to live in. Fertile mucus, which is less acid and less dense, is an ideal medium for sperm.

3. Mucus, which varies in color, thickness, amount, slipperiness and stretchability, can be felt on the

inner lips of the vagina or can be looked at by taking a sample from your vagina or cervix.

4. Mucus symptoms such as color, thickness, amount, etc. tell you when to stop having intercourse BEFORE ovulation occurs. This symptom, along with several others, corroborates BBT findings, and can be used in special instances when BBT is not accurate (fever, menopause, breast-feeding).

5. Statistically, the period is a safe time for most women. But careful observation and an analysis of YOUR cycle must be made to determine if it is safe for YOU!!!

CHAPTER FIVE

Learning to Recognize
Your Pattern of Fertility

The purpose of this chapter is to introduce program users to a variety of temperature patterns and mucus changes. Although we cannot predict what your graph or chart will look like, we can offer a selection of graphs and charts illustrating a number of situations that can occur while using the program. We encourage you to take the time to read the discussion of the graph's interpretation while you look at the graph. Hopefully, it will make you more comfortable interpreting your own graphs.

The first few graphs illustrate variations in length of cycle and time of ovulation. Other sample graphs include a graph with artifact readings; a graph with no progesterone rise (monophasic curve); a graph from someone recently off oral contraceptives; and graphs with readings that might be misinterpreted. We conclude with graphs illustrating special situations where BBT is not helpful (menopause and breast-feeding). All graphs include observations of mucus changes and various other observations the women have made.

After studying these sample graphs, you will be ready to interpret your own. By the time you have charted the recommended six months of cycles yourself, you should be confident in your ability to know when you are safe to have intercourse without risking pregnancy.

Artifact Readings

Look at Figure 14. First notice that the entire cycle for this woman is 30 days long. She started her next period on Day 31. Next notice that she has x'ed out the days (1 through 5) when she was having her menstrual flow. You can take your temperature during your period if you want. Chris did in the beginning. It might be useful in the first months of observations, but it is not necessary. The temperature during menses, which is

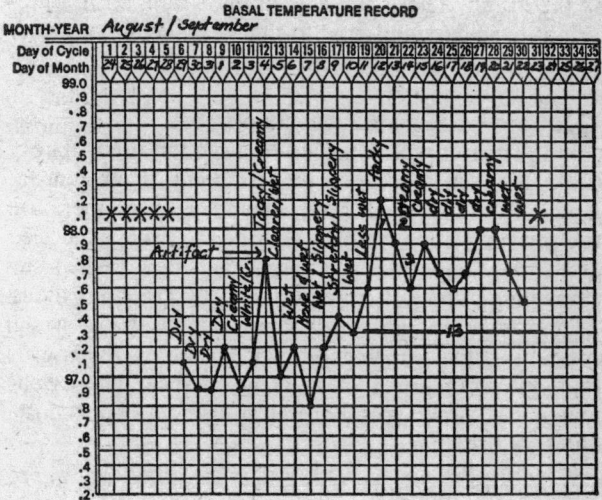

Figure 14 A temperature graph showing the mucus cycle and an artifact on day twelve.

higher at first, gradually lowers to the preovulatory baseline level and is not significant in determining the fertile time of your cycle. The exception to this rule is the woman who ovulates very early. (See page 48, "Deciding on Safety During Menses," for more discussion of this case.)

In Figure 14, the first temperature, 97.1 is taken on Day 6, the 29th of August. It remains within a close baseline temperature range until Day 12, when it rises sharply to 97.8. Since it drops way back to the preovulatory level on Day 13, and remains down for several days, we can determine that the reading on Day 12 was not a significant reading. This is called an artifact: a recording on the graph that seems out of line with the expected reading. It is not to be ignored. Indeed, it is duly recorded on the graph. One should just keep in mind that it seems out of place when interpreting the graph. These artifacts are not rare, so it is important to understand how to interpret them—or, more importantly, how to avoid misinterpreting them.

What Causes a Sudden Preovulatory Rise

Many factors can be involved in a sudden preovulatory rise: a low grade fever, a restless night, awakening at an unusual (for you) hour, taking your temperature after dashing to a child's bedside. We have noticed that Chris' temperature varies up and down when she is traveling. We just note this on the graph to avoid misinterpretation. Circumstances such as these which result in artifact readings do not invalidate the use of graph interpretation. There is no chance that we or anyone else would misinterpret an artifact as the postovulatory rise:

First, because we know that we must wait to see the *sustained rise for three days;*

Second, because we use mucus symptoms to corroborate our findings and the mucus symptom would indicate either fertile or prefertile mucus present.

Determining When Ovulation Has Occurred

Now, moving further into the cycle, notice that between Day 18 and Day 20, there is a NET TEMPERATURE RISE OF 0.9 degree. After Day 20, the temperature dips slightly, sort of bobbing up and down, but it remains essentially within a baseline that is significantly higher than the preovulatory baseline of this biphasic curve. The average temperature between Days 6 and 18 is 97.1 (even counting the artifact reading). The average temperature between Days 19 and 30 is about 97.8. This is an average difference of 0.7 degree. It is this NET DIFFERENCE, this TWO-PHASED CURVE, this DIFFERENCE IN BASELINES, that represents the pre- and postovulatory times. Since the dip before the rise indicates ovulation, we can see that this woman ovulated on Day 18. She was within a postovulatory safe period on Day 22 (since she could not be sure Day 19 was part of the rise she waited until Day 22 before having unprotected intercourse, counting Days 20, 21 and 22 as the "rise" days).

It is very important to understand the difference between the NET RISE and the individual dips and peaks of the graph. It would be simple if our recordings were always consistent: one temperature before ovulation, a single dip at the time of ovulation, and another even temperature (straight line on the graph) after ovulation. But, this is not the case. There is, however, this net difference in baselines, discernible by looking at the graph or averaging the temperatures.

Again, look at the graph. Notice that although the temperature dipped from Day 21 at 97.9 to 97.6 on Day 22, the Day 22 recording is still clearly higher than any of the preovulatory readings (this excludes the Day 13 reading, which is clearly "off the charts").

Looking at Day 15, you might wonder why this was not the ovulation point. Notice that in the three days following Day 15, the temperature still remains within a general preovulatory range. After Day 18, which we

pinpointed as ovulation, the rise is PRONOUNCED
AND MOVES INTO ANOTHER TEMPERATURE
BASELINE ALTOGETHER. Again, this is what we
are looking for when interpreting BBT readings.

Mucus Method
Note that using the mucus method, Figure 14 indicates
"dry days" from Day 6 to Day 9 of this cycle. Assuming that a woman has determined her menses to be
safe, unprotected intercourse would be possible from
Day 1 to Day 9. On Day 10 the first mucus symptom
appears: the creamy, tacky, white mucus that researchers feel may be infertile mucus. To be on the safe side
unprotected intercourse should stop WHEN THE
FIRST MUCUS SYMPTOM APPEARS. On Day 13,
the mucus thinned out, became more clear and is described as "wet" until the peak symptom on Day 17
when the mucus shows the spinnbarkeit symptom of
stretchability. On ovulation Day 18, mucus remains
"wet," but decreases on Day 19, returning first to tacky
and then to dry. Just before the period, a wet symptom
is noted again, but since fertility for that cycle has
ended unprotected intercourse is safe.

When was this woman safe? As we said, she could
have sex from Day 1 to Day 9. She resumed unprotected intercourse on Day 22 until Day 30. This is 17
"safe" days and 13 "unsafe" (potentially fertile) days
in a 30 day cycle.

At the end of a cycle you can often calculate the day
of ovulation by counting backwards. Menstruation usually starts about two weeks (14 days) after ovulation.
As you see, this woman had her period 13 days after
Day 18. This, of course, in no way helps with contraception, but can be helpful in determining the safety of
intercourse during menses, and is another example of
the regular rhythm of each woman's cycle.

Pronounced Biphasic Curve

Figure 15 shows a very dramatic biphasic curve. Menses occurs between Days 1 and 5. From Day 6 to Day 13 the average temperature is 97.2. On Day 14 the temperature rises to 97.8, on Day 15 to 98.0 and on Day 16 to 98.1. During the second half of this cycle, when progesterone was raising the woman's temperature, the BBT averaged 98.0. Although the initial rise from Day 13 to Day 14 was only 0.5 degree, the continual rise for the next two days indicates that the Day 14 reading represents the beginning of the progesterone (nonfertile) part of the cycle. This correct

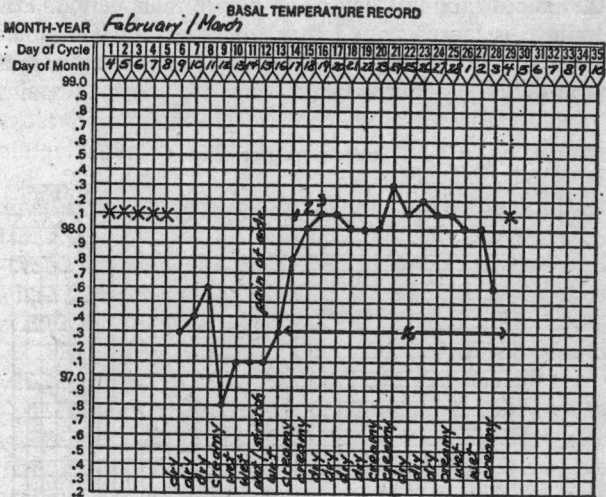

Figure 15 A pronounced biphasic curve.

assumption was reinforced by mucus observation. The wettest, stretchiest mucus is noted on Day 12, the day before ovulation. She also noted a pain on her right side on Day 12. This was probably the mittelschmertz symptom.

Counting Day 14 as the first day of the sustained rise, intercourse would be safe on Day 16. When you first start the program you may tend to be cautious and wait until Day 17 to be sure. That's fine. Caution is advised with the program. But as you watch your cycles month after month, you will become more secure in your knowledge and observations.

One other note on this sample chart. You will notice that on Day 28, there is a significant dip in temperature to 97.6. Such a dip at this point in the cycle is no need for concern. It in no way indicates the possibility of another ovulation. This is not biologically possible. But many women report that they notice the temperature dip on the last day or so before their period. For some it is more marked than for others. If it is noteworthy in your graph, it can be a good indication that your period is about to begin.

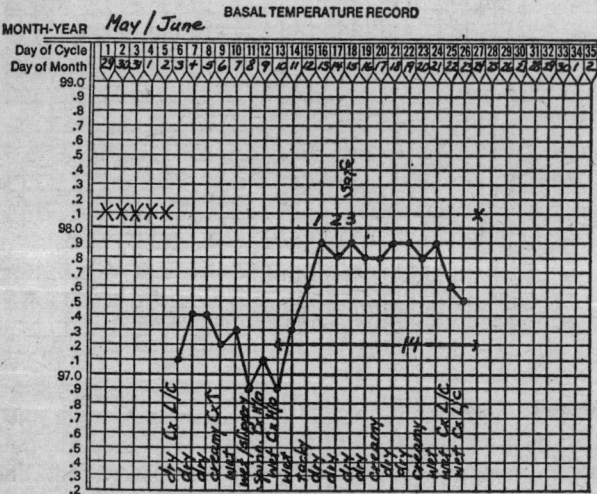

Figure 16 A gradual temperature rise.

A Gradual Temperature Rise

Figure 16 illustrates a gradual rise in temperature. Following a five day menstrual flow, from Day 6 to Day 13, the temperatures are pretty low, with a baseline of 97.2. On Day 14, the temperature rose to 97.3. This is not a 0.6 degree rise and further investigation is necessary. Mucus and cervix symptoms indicate that peak fertility is occurring, but they in no way indicate that it has passed.

On Day 15 the temperature is 97.6. This temperature is higher than any other for the cycle. This fact, coupled with the time of the month it is occurring, would tend to make you think that the progesterone portion of the cycle is in progress. However, since the rise is gradual, these assumptions, however reasonable, must not be relied upon. (Remember, progesterone makes the temperature rise and creates the nonfertile environment). On Day 16 we see that the temperature remains up and is in fact higher, at 97.9. To be on the safe side, we must count Day 16 as the first day of the rise. Therefore, on Day 18, sexual intercourse is safe without protection. Again, this is reinforced by mucus observations which show that the mucus gradually decreased in wetness from Days 13 and 14 until the vagina felt "dry" again.

It is important to understand with a chart like this one that although you can clearly see IN RETROSPECT that ovulation occurred on Day 13 (menstruation started exactly two weeks later) and that intercourse was safe on Day 16, THIS WAS NOT AT ALL CLEAR ON DAY 16 due to the gradual rise.

This woman uses cervical observations as well as temperature and mucus symptoms. She noted the cervix was low and closed after her period, high and opened around the time of ovulation. She further noted that it lowered and closed so that it was quite low in the vagina again at the time of her next period.

Combining all of these observations is what makes

the program work. This woman was free to have unprotected intercourse from Days 1 to 8 and again from
Day 18 to Day 28. This totals 10 fertile and 17 nonfertile days in a 26 day cycle.

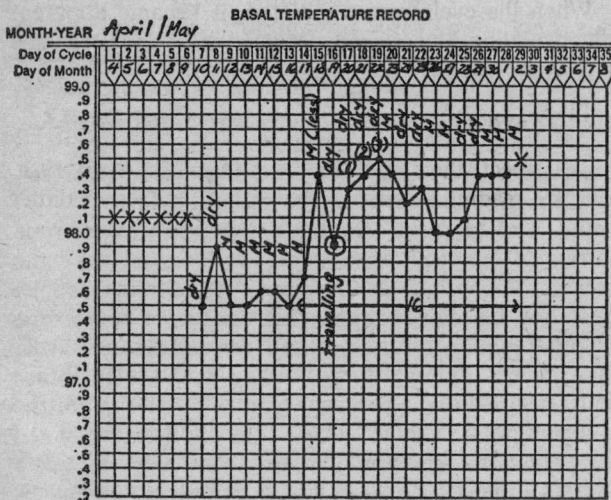

Figure 17 This graph shows an artifact on day sixteen. Although in
retrospect it's apparent that ovulation did occur on day 13, this
woman waited three more days before resuming unprotected intercourse, to be absolutely certain.

An Artifact Around the Time of Ovulation

Figure 17 represents another graph with an artifact, or
reading that seems out of line with what one would
expect. The 28 day cycle starts with a 6 day period.
From Day 7 to Day 13, temperatures remain relatively
low, with a baseline of 97.6. As you see, there was a
rise on Days 14 and 15 of 0.2 and 0.7 degrees re-
spectively. She might have thought that this represented
her postovulatory rise, but then on Day 16, the temperature dropped to 97.9. A notation beside the tem-

perature indicates that she was traveling. This *might* have affected her temperature.

> *But, to be certain, she waited until Day 19 to resume unprotected sexual intercourse.*

When the cycle was completed, it became apparent that ovulation had indeed occurred on Day 13 as she had suspected, but

> *this was not apparent until three days after Day 13.*

In retrospect, then, she could see that the April 19th, Day 16, reading was somewhat of an artifact. It didn't really "jibe" with the rest of the biphasic curve.

This fact was further supported by mucus observation. This woman chooses to note only dry or wet days, rather than all of the various changes in between. If it is a dry day, she considers it safe, if it is wet *at all* and before her temperature rise, she considers it unsafe. After dry days on Days 7 and 8, she recorded a mucus symptom until Day 16. Then she noted dry days on Day 16 through 19. If Day 16 was the ovulation day, she would have had a mucus symptom, that is, felt that sensation of wetness.

You'll notice that this woman has some wet days after ovulation. This does occur, but does not indicate an early fertility sign as it would if it occurred before ovulation. Most women say that although they may feel wet after ovulation, it is not the same thin, lubricative, stretchy mucus of preovulatory days.

Allowing for extra days for the artifact, this woman had an 11 day period where unprotected intercourse was inadvisable and an 18 day period which she considered to be safe.

The Irregular Cycle
Figure 18 represents the so-called "irregular" cycle. This cycle occurred for Chris after many "regular," 28 day cycles. It was a variation for her, but posed no

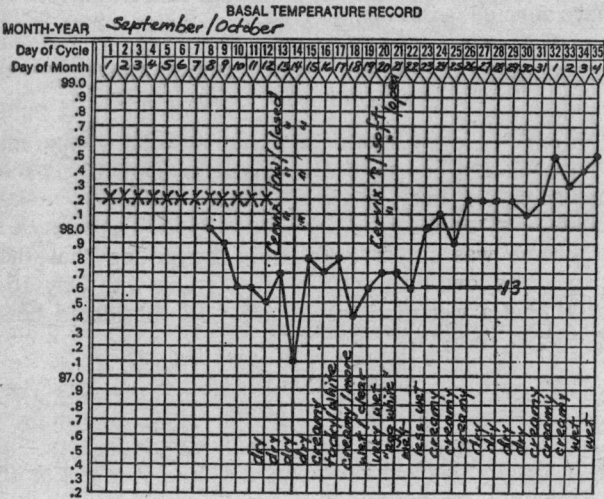

Figure 18 An irregular cycle with ovulation on day 22.

safety threat, since, with this program, each cycle is viewed individually.

To begin with, there was an unusually long menses, from Day 1 to Day 12. Since this pattern was unusual, Chris began taking her temperature on Day 8 of the period. She noted that it lowered gradually during the last part of the period. This is a common temperature manifestation of the change from the menstrual or shedding phase to the proliferative or growing phase of the cycle (what is being "shed" or "grown" is the endometrium or lining of the uterus.)

Notice that from Day 13 (after her period) to Day 22, the temperature baseline is 97.6. From Day 23 to 35, the temperature baseline rises to 98.2. This is, of course, a net rise of 0.6 degrees. She ovulated on Day 22 (notice that her period came 13 days later), but this was not apparent at first. She had a good rise on Days 23 and 24, but then a dip on Day 25 to within the preovulatory baseline made her uncertain about the safety of that period. So, she started to count "rise days" with Day 26. The first day she considered safe was Day 28.

Chris considered the first six days of the cycle as a safe period. Then, when the period continued, she became suspicious, considered herself unsafe and started recording her BBT. When the period ended she noted definite dry days from Day 12 to Day 15. The safety of this time was further confirmed by noting that the cervix was low, firm and closed. Starting with Day 16, she noted a wet mucus symptom and considered herself fertile until Day 28.

With the confusion caused by this variation cycle, Chris lost some safe days. For this cycle she considered herself safe on 18 days of the 35 day cycle. We included this cycle because such "unusual" patterns can occur. They may decrease "safe" days, but they do not decrease the safety of the program.

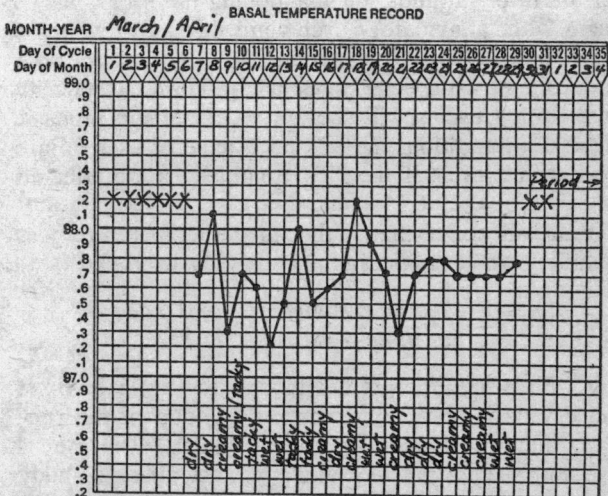

Figure 19 A monophasic cycle.

Monophasic Curve: No Definite Rise
Figure 19 is an example of a cycle that has no definitive rise because of little or no evidence of progesterone (the hormone that causes the temperature rise). Although these cycles usually indicate that the woman did not ovulate, one cannot assume that intercourse is safe with such a pattern for two reasons:

First, a woman can ovulate and not show the characteristic biphasic curve. This is by far the exception to the rule, but it can happen.

Second, you cannot know until after the fact that the cycle was anovulatory (without ovulation occurring).

Remember, the New Birth Control Program cannot predict ovulation.

The occurrence of a cycle like this one is not cause for alarm or grounds for abandoning the program. To begin with, anovulatory cycles are unusual if you are not breast-feeding or experiencing menopause (more about these two special times later). The vast majority of recorded cycles will show a characteristic biphasic pattern. In addition, there is no chance of user failure with such a cycle if the NBCP guidelines are adhered to.

You will notice that, although the temperature goes up and down (as high as 98.2 and as low as 97.3),

it never reflects a sustained rise of 0.6 degrees for three consecutive days.

You will also notice that although the cycle has wet and dry days, there is no marked buildup of the slippery, thinner, stretchy, egg white mucus. The mucus symptom seems "patchy," and *is,* in fact, since the body is never really preparing to ovulate.

Some women feel that the mucus method can be

used alone with such cycles to tell you when you can and cannot have sexual intercourse. The mucus symptom is very helpful, but we recommend that program users combine BBT readings and mucus observations for greatest safety. In this way, the mucus symptom will tell you when to stop unprotected intercourse, and the BBT will tell you when to resume intercourse after ovulation has occurred for the cycle. If you are breast-feeding or experiencing menopause, you will need to rely on the mucus symptom more heavily. But, for the occasional monophasic cycle, we recommend combined use of both symptoms.

A monophasic cycle necessitates abstinence from sexual intercourse or use of a diaphragm or condom (with their inherent safety risks) in order to prevent pregnancy.

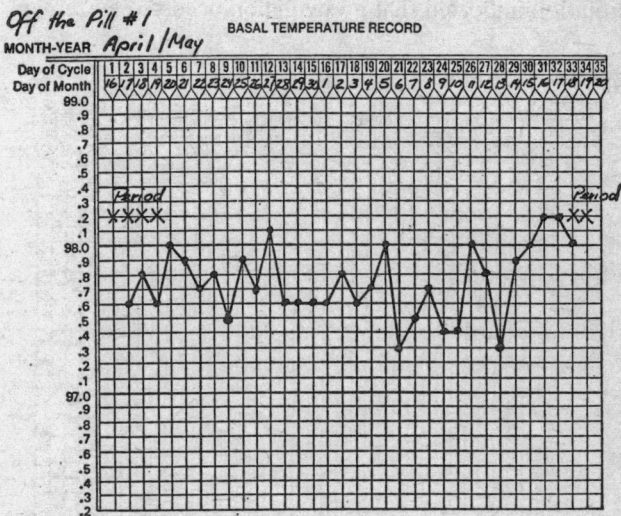

Figure 20

Coming Off the Pill

One woman who attended a course on the use of the program was taking oral contraceptives (pills). After learning about this new way to understand her fertility, she decided to stop taking the pill. Figures, 20, 21, 22 and 23 show the temperature patterns that this woman had for the first four cycles that she was off the pill.

As you can see, for the first three months, she had a monophasic curve. It was like the anovulatory curve mentioned above but with more extremes of temperature changes.

She seemed to have developed a somewhat biphasic curve in Figure 22, but ovulation was uncertain because of the dips on Days 24 and 25 and again on Days 32 and 33. She felt that mucus symptom interpretation indicated that no ovulation occurred since her

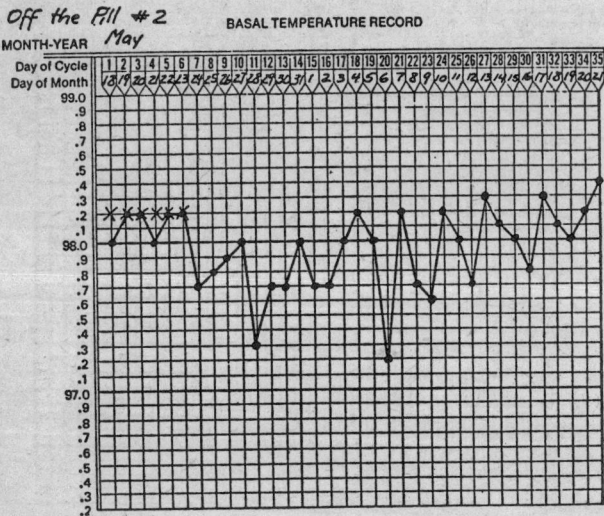

Figure 21

mucus secretions went back and forth from tacky and white to dry, never reaching the fertile, preovulatory stage.

Finally, four months after going off the pill (she was only *on* the pill for five months!) her curve was clearly biphasic (see Figure 23). After a four day period, with the exception of the Day 8 artifact due to illness, her temperature remained low until Day 23. Along with this "normal" preovulatory baseline, she experienced a buildup of fertile mucus which peaked on Days 21 and 22.

On Day 24, the temperature rose 0.3 degree. By Day 25, the temperature was much higher than elsewhere in the cycle and remained up until her next period started. Counting Day 25 as the first day of the rise, she was safe to have unprotected intercourse on Day 27. With the dry days in the beginning of the cycle, she had 15 safe days in this 33 day cycle.

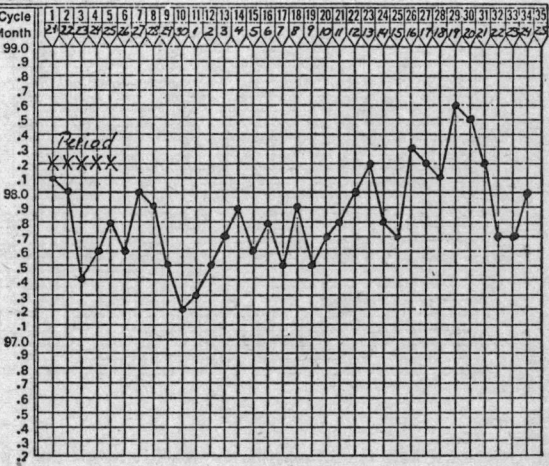

Figure 22

The Weekend Syndrome

This next figure, 24, illustrates what happens when you vary temperature taking time on a regular basis. If you get up every weekday morning at 7:00 a.m. and then sleep in on Saturday and Sunday mornings to 10:00 or 11:00, you may get a graph that shows little plateaus where the weekends occur. We think of 7:00 and 11:00 as "morning" but the three to four hour difference can make a difference in your reading. It seems to be more pronounced for some women than for others. We have noted it from time to time on Chris' charts.

On this graph of Chris' (Figure 24), weekends occurred noticeably on Days 9 and 10 and Days 16 and

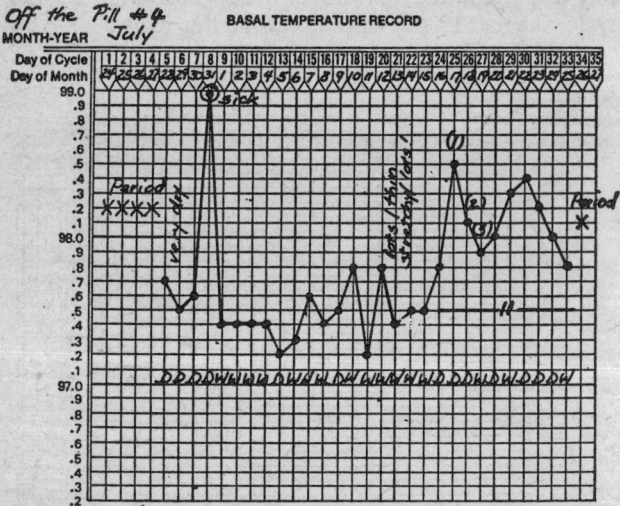

Figure 23

Figures 20-23 These four graphs show a woman's temperature patterns for her first four cycles after coming off the pill.

17. The first plateau is preovulatory. There is no way that we would have mistaken it for the rise because it was not sustained for three days, and it was not elevated enough. The second plateau (Days 16 and 17) looked like part of the postovulatory rise. It was, just elevated a little higher. While the temperature looked like it dropped on Day 18, we didn't take that as a sign that ovulation had not occurred yet, because although it was a lower temperature, it was well within the postovulatory baseline.

We mention this weekend syndrome, not because it can cause gross misinterpretation of the graph, but because understanding its existence can help explain graphs that appear to be very choppy. If you are getting up at various times during the week, it might be a good idea to note this on your graph, to facilitate its interpretation.

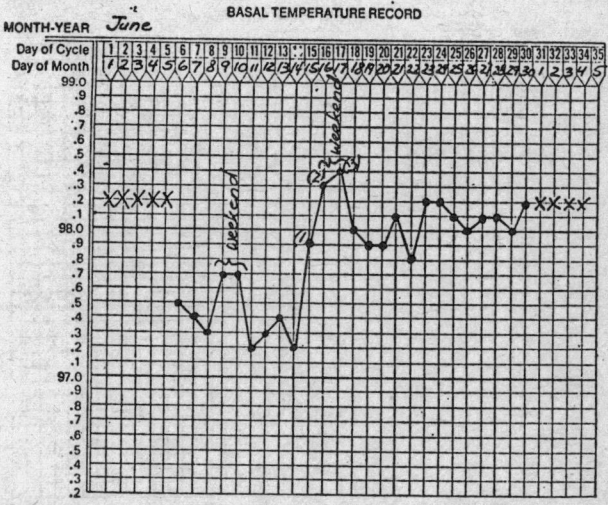

Figure 24 A graph showing two examples of the "weekend syndrome."

Another Monophasic Curve: Breast-feeding and Menopause

There are times in every woman's life when ovulation does not occur. We have already mentioned the occasional anovulatory cycle. In addition, breast-feeding and the menopausal transition may result in times when it is not useful to observe temperature patterns to delineate fertile periods.

When a woman is breast-feeding her baby, she MAY not ovulate for several months after the baby is born. This is never a certainty, however, and women are cautioned not to use breast-feeding as a method of birth control. If you are breast-feeding and waiting for your first period to worry about contraception, remember that the period comes 14 days AFTER the ovulation. So you will ovulate and be fertile BEFORE your period comes.

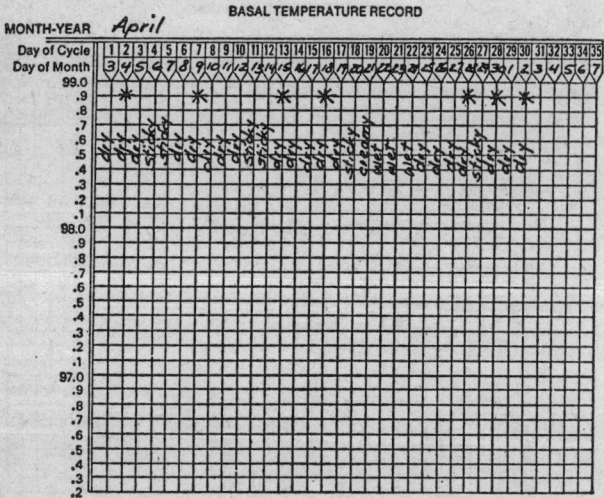

Figure 25 A mucus observation chart of a breast-feeding woman. The asterisks indicate days when she had intercourse.

A similar situation confronts the woman who is going through menopause. She may not ovulate for several cycles, but until she has completely stopped menstruating, she cannot be sure that she will not ovulate again.

Both groups of women cannot rely on temperature readings and both need reliable contraception. For these women, we recommend carefully observed and cautiously applied use of the Mucus Method combined with observations of mittelschmertz and midcycle spotting. Noting the position of the cervix as described in Chapter Four can be helpful as well. Since these instances require heavy reliance on the Mucus Method, we do not recommend use of this for contraception if you have never used the entire program prior to starting to breast-feed or reaching menopause. We feel that you need some experience with using the combined methods before applying mucus observations alone.

A record should be kept of mucus changes. Figure 25 shows one way to organize a mucus observation chart. In the same way as you did while taking temperature readings, you would observe mucus at about the same time every day, recording the type of mucus you observe. You would also note other relevant symptoms.

Several Rules for Finding the Safe Periods During Menopause and While Breast-feeding

1. Definitely dry days are safe for unprotected intercourse.

2. Abstain the day of any mucus symptom. Abstain for one additional day if the mucus was the early, sticky, flaky, white type. Watch to see if the mucus symptom changes.

3. Abstain for three days after the cessation of any fertile mucus symptom (wet, lubricative,

stretchy, egg white). Intercourse is safe on the fourth day after the cessation of such mucus.

4. Make sure that any bleeding that you have is menstrual bleeding and not ovulatory, mid-cycle spotting. Confirm that you definitely have a flow before figuring that it is a safe period.

5. If you have any doubts about whether or not a mucus symptom is fertile, assume it is fertile and wait that day and three days after it stops to have intercourse.

This last rule is perhaps the most important one to follow. Women who have used the mucus symptom for a long time claim that they can differentiate the sticky, tacky mucus from the fertile, wet, mucus. Researchers currently believe that the sticky, white, curdled mucus is *probably* not fertile. Most women who use this method alone agree with this finding. However, to feel more secure, you should not have intercourse with any mucus symptom.

One more caution. We have stated all along that the program involved BBT as well as mucus observation for optimal safety and accuracy. Since we believe this to be true, you would be decreasing the safety factor to some degree by using mucus observation alone. Many women have used mucus alone with success when breast-feeding. We encourage the very strictest adherence to the rules for greatest safety.

A Mucus Observation Chart

If you choose to use mucus observation alone during menopause or breast-feeding, Figure 25 will give you an idea of how mucus recording looks and is interpreted. It represents part of a record of a woman who has breast-fed her baby for two months. On Days 1 through 3 she notes a definite dryness, so she is safe to have unprotected intercourse. The asterisks indicate days when she had intercourse. After having sexual relations on Day 2, she abstained on Day 3, even though she was still dry. She wanted to make sure she would not mistake semen for a wet symptom or vice versa. This is a good policy in the beginning, as a safety precaution.

Since the sticky mucus appeared on Days 4 and 5, she abstained until Day 7, when the dry symptom was clearly present again.

Now, notice that from Day 18 to Day 22, she experienced a buildup of fertile mucus. The symptom was at its peak on Day 22. She needed to wait until four days past this symptom to have intercourse. The symptom occurred on Day 22, so she was safe to have unprotected intercourse on Day 26. Notice that in the meantime, from Day 22 to 26, there was no recurrence of any mucus symptom. Such a recurrence would have necessitated further abstinence.

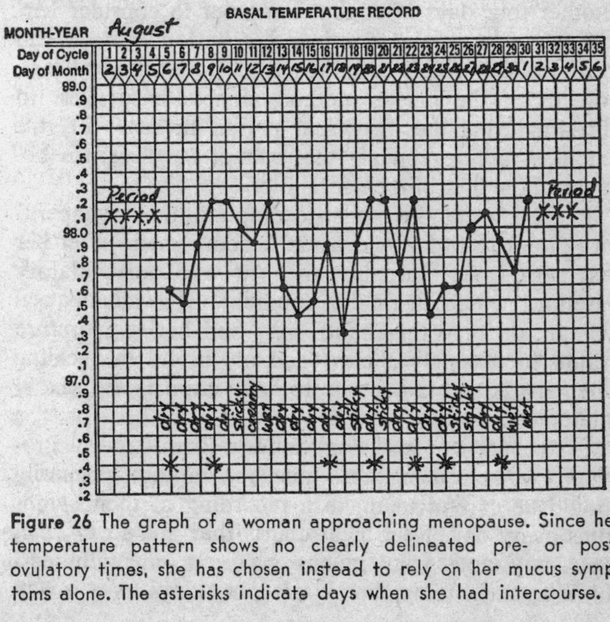

Figure 26 The graph of a woman approaching menopause. Since her temperature pattern shows no clearly delineated pre- or post-ovulatory times, she has chosen instead to rely on her mucus symptoms alone. The asterisks indicate days when she had intercourse.

Figure 26 is the temperature graph of a woman who is approaching menopause. As you can see, her temperature pattern is of no use to her here. It fluctuates up and down with no clearly delineated pre- and postovulatory times. She, therefore, has chosen to rely on her mucus symptom alone for determining fertility.

After a four day period (remember, menses does not necessarily cease because ovulation ceases), this woman experienced five dry days. She used these times for safe unprotected intercourse. Again, she waited after each intercourse day to make sure she was not confusing semen with wet mucus. From Day 10 to Day 12, she had a brief "patch" of mucus. It was not present for long, but this does not matter when calculating safe times. To be safe, she waited until the fourth day after the mucus symptom before having sexual intercourse again. Just before her next period, she experienced some wet days, and would have counted another four days after that symptom to consider herself safe. She cannot consider her period safe, as can most women with a definitive BBT pattern. Most proponents of the mucus method alone advise users to abstain during the menstrual period in case a fertile mucus symptom appears that cannot be discerned because of the flow of menstrual blood.

In the case of the breast-feeding mother, a temperature graph record would again become useful after her first period. At that time, the pre- and postovulatory baselines would again be apparent. The menopausal woman, on the other hand, may find her temperature graphs increasingly choppy and not useful in deciding when she is and is not safe to have unprotected sexual intercourse.

Like every woman using the New Birth Control Program, women using the mucus symptom primarily should be careful to make a recording of their symptoms every day. Keep neat charts that are up to date. You may note your mucus symptom mentally and think you will remember it later, but days have a way of slipping by unnoted. This can prove extremely hazardous.

Review

We hope that this section on graphs and charts has proved useful. As you begin keeping your own charts, refer back to this section from time to time. It will all make a lot more sense when you can relate the patterns and curves to symptoms you have observed in your own cycle. We still get an occasional pattern that is not what we would expect, but by adhering strictly to the rules of the program, we are always confident that we are not risking an unplanned pregnancy. Remember:

REMEMBER:

1. It is observation of the mucus symptom that tells you when to stop having intercourse in your cycle.

2. It is observation of the 0.6 degree temperature rise for three consecutive days that tells you when to resume having intercourse after ovulation has occurred.

3. Patterns in temperature vary, but most (monophasic curves being the rare exception) shows pre- and postovulatory baselines that can be observed and interpreted by you.

4. Some graphs show "out of line" very high or very low readings called artifacts. These should be recorded and noted including any unusual circumstances (e.g. fever, stress, etc.)

5. A monophasic, "no rise" curve may occur occasionally and necessitates abstinence or use of contraceptive devices for that cycle.

6. For women who are menopausal or breast-feeding, the mucus method alone may be used with extreme caution and strict adherence to the rules. Safety is somewhat decreased when the mucus method is used alone.

CHAPTER SIX

Anatomy and Physiology

Many of us are reluctant to discuss our bodies and especially hesitant to learn more about our reproductive organs. This feeling was probably initiated when we were young and asked our parents embarrassing questions about the "facts of life." Then it was reinforced by dull, never-to-the-point high school biology classes in which there wasn't a living connection between anatomy and physiology and our own bodies. And if we weren't discouraged by our schools, family and peers some of us were likely alienated by some medical person's oneupmanship. For example:

You: Doctor, I have noticed a small lump on my cervix and wondered if I could have a cervical erosion?

Doctor: This without accompanying clinical findings and history is meaningless. Have you had an increase in leukorrhea, noticed increased mittleschmertz pain, had a prolonged dysmenorrhea with menses? Has anyone ever told you that your uterus is retroverted? Do you often examine your own cervix?

This may sound somewhat exaggerated, but the situation is more than likely recognizable. In any case, if you have felt discouraged, alienated or put off by your own anatomy, this chapter will provide you with a simple look at the beauty and intricacy of your femaleness. We recommend it for men, too. Knowing your body is a wonderful part of knowing yourself and it makes the

New Birth Control Program that much more interesting and understandable.

So, if you have had a difficult time in the past, try this one more time.

1. Look at the diagrams and illustrations while you read the chapter. If you can study it with a friend, you'll probably like doing it that much more. If you have a friend to do it with, have the friend read the text while you pick out the parts in the pictures.

2. Say the words out loud so you'll remember them and be able to use them again.

3. Remember that the pictures in the drawings are really parts of your body. Don't be afraid to touch the parts on yourself. That way their position and size will be that much more understandable.

You can probably use the NBCP with a minimal knowledge of anatomy but the program will take on a much fuller meaning if you understand the parts and the process. When you begin to correlate the changes in your mucus and temperature with the cycle, the importance of the anatomy and physiology will become more apparent.

Uterus

In the center of Figure 27 is a pear-shaped structure. This is the uterus or womb. It is about the size of your fist (2 to 3 inches) and fits down low in the abdomen behind your pubic bone. It is an amazing organ because it can stretch 518 times that size to accommodate a baby. Then, when the baby is born, it returns to pretty much the same size as before the pregnancy.

Notice that the uterus is divided into two parts. The top part is called the fundus and it is about two thirds of the uterus. The bottom part is called the cervix. The cervix plays a significant role in the New Birth Control Program because it goes through dynamic changes during the menstrual cycle.

First of all, you will notice that the cervix is open at

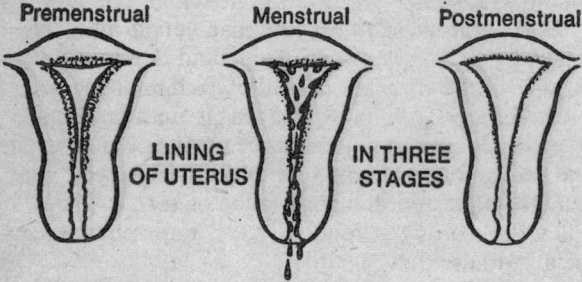

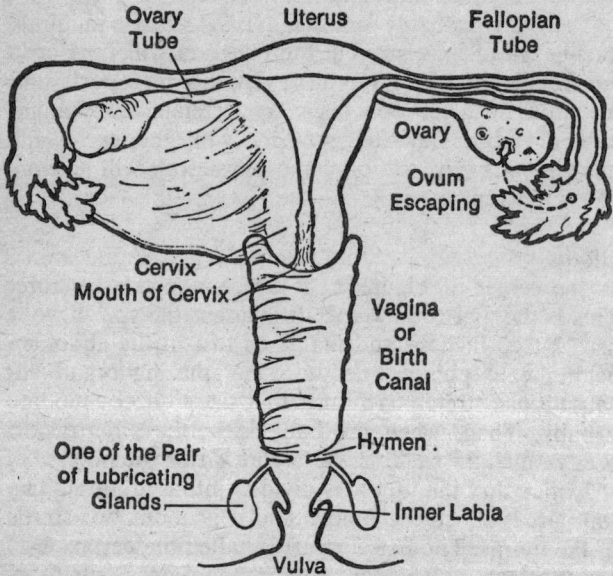

Figure 27 The female reproductive organs.

the bottom end. This opening, called the os, is the place through which sperm swim to enter the uterus after intercourse and ejaculation. The cervix also contains small glands that secrete some fluid that runs into the vagina. The amount and kind of fluid changes with your changing fertility cycle and makes up a large part of your normal vaginal discharge. Some discharge is natural and can be used to determine when you are fertile. It is called *mucus*.

Ovaries

Look back at Figure 27 again. Notice that to the right and left of the uterus are two tubelike organs. These are the fallopian tubes. They are the passageway for the egg to travel from the ovary to the uterus. At the ends of the fallopian tubes are two rounded structures. These organs are the ovaries, and they contain the eggs that are released each month when you ovulate. Actually about 250,000 of these eggs are in the ovaries at the time of birth. They remain dormant in the ovaries until puberty and then begin the natural cycle of development and death that goes along with the changes in your natural fertile cycle.

The process of maturation of the egg continues on a regular basis from puberty until menopause. Some months you won't ovulate even though you have a period. However, most months one egg, which lives for 12 to 36 hours, is released, with the right and left ovaries alternating each month. Unless, of course, you are taking oral contraceptives. Then, the pill provides you with hormones that act to shut down the process of ovulation by making your body think that it has already ovulated.

As the time for ovulation (production of the egg) approaches a blisterlike bump forms on the outside of the ovary. This blister gets bigger and bigger until it bursts open, releasing the egg. The egg then enters the fallopian tube, where it can meet the approaching sperm. If you look in Figure 28 you can see that the

FERTILIZATION

Fallopian Tube

Ovary

Uterus   Route of sperm
                                    Route of ovum

Semen deposited in vagina

Vagina

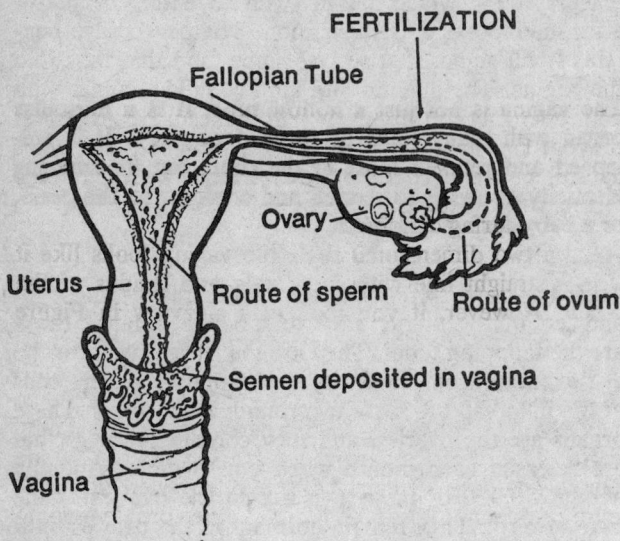

Figure 28 Fertilization

sperm can swim all the way up into the tubes to meet
with the egg. The meeting of the egg and sperm is fertilization.

Your ovaries are quite far down in the abdomen.
They are analogous to the male testes but are more
safely confined in the abdomen for protection. You
probably have never felt them with your hands, but
you may have felt them "no hands" if you have had a
cramping pain for a day or so around the middle of
your cycle. This midcycle or mittleschmertz pain is
caused by the pressure of the blister forming and burst-
ing, and many women can use this to detect ovulation.
Studies have shown that midcycle pain can occur just
prior to, during or just after ovulation, so it shouldn't
be used alone to detect ovulation. However, it is an

excellent way to add to the other observations that we have discussed—temperature, mucus, cervical positioning.

Vagina

The vagina is not just a hollow tube. It is a muscular organ with many folds or rugae (roo-gay). It is collapsed and relaxed most of the time, but its amazing elasticity allows it to stretch and conform to the penis, or a baby during childbirth.

On a two dimensional scale the vagina looks like it is in a straight line with the cervix and fundus of the uterus. However, if you look at a sideview in Figure 29 you will notice that the cervix and uterus are actually at right angles to each other. In about 70% of women the fundus is tipped forward (anteverted) while in the remaining 30% it is retroverted (tipped backward). Tipping backward is a normal variation of the female anatomy. Thus, having a retroverted uterus is not a problem unless there is some other problem going on that calls it to your attention.

Notice that the cervix enters the vagina at an angle also. This is important because the vagina and cervix are in a dynamic relationship that changes with your changing fertility cycle. Most of the time the cervix is low in the vagina and pointing backwards, towards the rectum. It is generally hard and closed also. As your body gets ready to ovulate the ligaments that are attached to the cervix contact, pulling it forward and upward in the vagina. At the same time it also softens and opens slightly (See "Other Noteworthy Changes" on page 45). These changes, as well as the glandular changes that we already mentioned in Chapter Four, prepare your body for ovulation. They change a woman's internal environment from one unfavorable for the life and movement of sperm to one in which sperm can live, swim and gain nutrients (energy supply).

A Word About Conception

It is important to relate the anatomical parts of a woman's body to the process of conception, to really understand the New Birth Control Program. Most of us know that pregnancy occurs when the sperm and egg unite. The sperm comes from the male sexual system, and pregnancy occurs when semen (sperm-filled fluid) from the penis is deposited in the vagina, and sperm

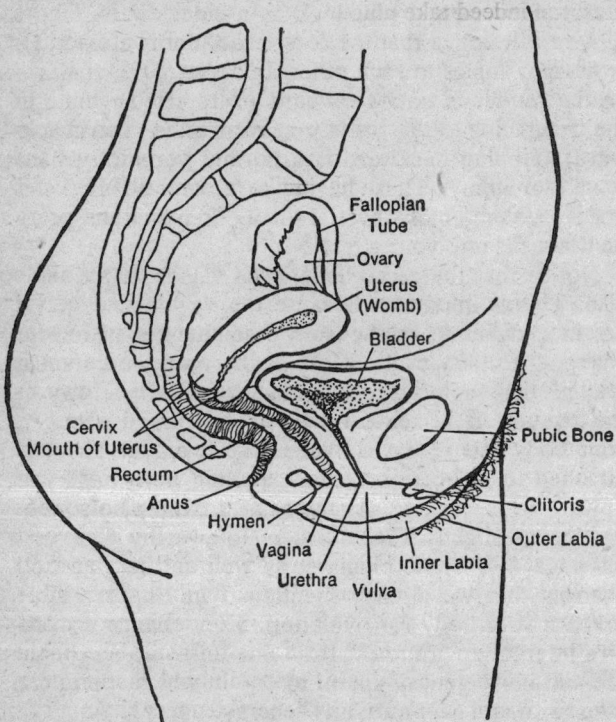

Figure 29 A side view of the female pelvic organs.

swim through the os (opening in the cervix), through the uterus and into the fallopian tubes. If the time is right, a single sperm can penetrate the egg and begin the process of creating a new human being.

We say that sperm is deposited, not to make love sound mechanical, but to emphasize that *penetration need not take place for conception to occur*. One ejaculation can contain up to 400,000 million sperm, and some sperm live in the fluid the male produces before he actually ejaculates. If any sperm are pushed into the vagina during mutual masturbation, foreplay or contraceptive "nearsies" (like withdrawal), pregnancy can indeed take place.

To relate this to the female anatomy that we have just described, you need to remember that the woman's reproductive system is essentially open. The vagina and the cervix are not firmly closed structures. Sperm can swim, and if they have entrance to the woman's genital tract they can move along it like a conduit. The end result is that carelessness is likely to result in pregnancy.

The External Anatomy

Looking at Figure 30 you will see the external female sexual organs or genitalia. Unlike the male, the female sexual organs are difficult to visualize. The best way to get to know this part of your body is to read about it, understand it and then look at it in real life. There is no taboo against looking at your own body. All you need is a hand mirror. Diagrams, no matter how true-to-life, just aren't the real thing.

First notice the outside oval of skin and hair around the vagina. The large lips, or labia majora, are visible without the mirror and serve as a fatty tissue protection for the genitals. A small oval exists inside the labia majora and it is called the labia minora. In this area are glands that secrete fluids during sexual excitement.

Now look at Figure 30 from top to bottom. First, from the top is the clitoris. The clitoris is the sensitive

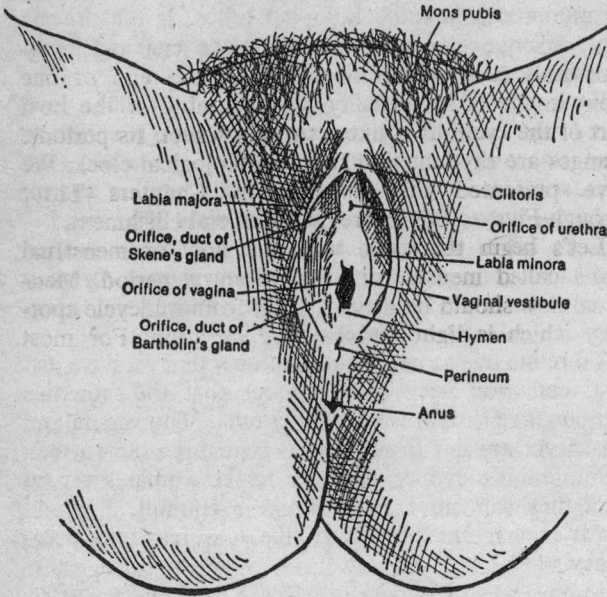

Figure 30 The external female sexual organs.

center of sexual excitement for the female. It is made up of spongy tissue that becomes erect and engorged with blood during sexual arousal. In an anatomical sense it is an analog of the man's penis, since both organs develop from the same tissue (source) in the embryo. The clitoris is covered by a protective hood called the prepuce.

The opening below the clitoris is the urethra (your-ree-thruh). It is the opening that connects with your bladder and allows urine to flow out of the body. The next larger opening is the vagina, which we have already described. And finally, the next opening below is the anus, or external opening of the bowel.

Mapping the Menstrual Cycle

The fertility cycle of a woman repeats itself on a regular basis each month or so. Thus, the end of one event in the cycle is really the beginning of the next part of the cycle. It is like a turning wheel. Its periodic changes are rhythms that follow a biological clock. We have presented this material in Chapters Three through Five, so this is a review with embellishment.

Let's begin the cycle with the flow of menstrual blood called menses, or more often, a period. Menstrual flow should be distinguished from midcycle spotting, which is light and brief in duration. For most women, the menstrual flow starts with pinkish red spotting, quickly increasing to a moderate or heavy discharge or dark red blood mixed with other secretions. The discharge is sufficient to warrant the use of a pad or tampon to absorb the flow. During this time, the lining of the uterus, called the endometrium, is shed.

On Day 6, the bloody discharge usually stops and the ovary begins to ready itself to release an egg into the fallopian tube adjacent to it. At the same time, the lining of the uterus gets thicker and richer in anticipation of the possible fertilized egg that would implant and develop into a human baby. On Day 14 in the woman's cycle, the egg is released. This is called ovulation. It generally takes about six days for the egg to travel down the tube and into the uterus. If the egg is to be fertilized, this will occur in the tube, and six days later the fertilized egg may attach itself to the wall of the uterus where it will grow. So, an egg released on Day 14 will pass through the uterus by Day 20.

If implantation (attachment to the uterus) does not occur, the egg will be passed out of the body with other secretions. Then the uterine lining, no longer needed for the attachment of the fertilized egg, will be shed again in the form of the next menstrual period. Thus, on Day 28 the nonpregnant woman will have a period and begin Day 1 of the next cycle. As you can see, using the menses as Day 1 of the cycle is only an agreed-upon convenience, for each cycle will continue to proceed in a rhythm like a turning wheel.

Regulation of the Fertility Cycle

The regulation of the human sexual system is controlled by chemicals called hormones. The signal to produce these hormones comes from the brain, or central nervous system, and the message is transmitted in the form of chemicals to the sexual organs of the body. The mystery of hormones and body regulation is a relatively new science that is beginning to offer an explanation of the intricacy of the female menstrual cycle. We are providing a simple description of this process, since it could take many volumes to describe what is already known about the subject.

The two principal hormones that we are concerned with are estrogen and progesterone. The first one, estrogen, is made by the ovary in a small substructure called the follicle. This hormone is responsible for what are called secondary sex characteristics. These traits, such as enlarged breasts, a relatively hairless face and body, and fatty deposits at certain places on the body, are due to the production of estrogen. The level of estrogen that women produce differentiates them from men.

In addition to giving us these female characteristics, estrogen effects the endometrium (lining of the uterus) in a very important way. Secretion of estrogen proceeds simultaneously with the enlargement and development of the egg, and causes the endometrium to grow. The growth of the endometrium begins near the end of the menses as a result of the increase in the body's level of estrogen. Both the thickness of the lining and the level of estrogen increase as the cycle moves towards ovulation.

Estrogen affects your vaginal secretions, which originate in the glands of the cervix as well. After your

Fertility Awareness:
your own record

with rules, reminders,
and a year's supply
of personal charts

REMINDERS FOR TEMPERATURE TAKING

1. Take your basal body temperature (BBT) each day as the first thing you do, before getting up and eating or drinking.
2. Make sure the thermometer is shaken down well, and that you leave it in for 5 minutes.
3. Record each BBT reading daily on your graph. Remember: missed readings can result in an inaccurate graph.

REMINDERS FOR MUCUS OBSERVATIONS

1. Observe your mucus symptom daily, and about the same time each day.
2. Observe the amount, consistency, color, stretchiness and slipperyness.
3. Record your observations daily on your temperature graph.
4. Also, note other symptoms such as the position, consistency and whether or not your cervix is open slightly, each day on your graph. Record mittelschmerz symptom if you feel it.

HOW TEMPERATURE TELLS YOU WHEN YOU ARE FERTILE

1. Your preovulatory temperature will be lower than your temperature after ovulation.
2. At ovulation your temperature **may** show a slight dip if you take your temperature within a few hours of ovulation.
3. After ovulation your temperature will rise and

remain up until your next menstrual period.

4. ESSENTIAL RULE: After your temperature has gone up 0.6°F and stayed up there for three successive days, you are safe to have unprotected intercourse.

HOW MUCUS TELLS YOU WHEN YOU ARE FERTILE

1. Infertile mucus (really the absence of mucus, or a "dry" feeling on the lips of the vagina and on the cervical os) is too dense and too acid for sperm to live in.

2. Fertile mucus is an ideal medium for sperm to live. It is egg white in color, stretchy and slippery.

3. After your period you will have several "dry" days followed by an increase in fertile mucus that peaks just prior to ovulation.

4. After ovulation your mucus decreases, becoming less stretchy, more tacky and cloudier. Most importantly, it will decrease in amount.

5. ESSENTIAL RULE: When mucus is present it is unsafe to have unprotected intercourse. Remember that sperm can live in fertile mucus up to five days. Look ahead to be safe.

FERTILE MUCUS	NONFERTILE MUCUS
EGG WHITE CLEAR	CLOUDY
STRETCHY	NOT STRETCHY
SLIPPERY	TACKY-STICKY
COPIOUS	SCANT

HOW YOUR CERVIX CHANGES
DURING YOUR CYCLE

NON OVULATORY	OVULATORY
FIRM—LIKE YOUR NOSE	SOFT—LIKE YOUR LIPS
LOW IN THE VAGINA	HIGHER IN THE VAGINA
CLOSED	SLIGHTLY OPEN
DRY	MOIST

POSSIBLE PITFALLS

1. Take six full cycles of observations before using this method of fertility control. If you are unfamiliar with the method you are taking a serious chance.

2. Carefully consider whether or not your period is a "safe" time. For some women, menstrual bleeding will cover up their mucus symptom making it possible to become pregnant.

3. Don't ever try to predict the future. You must follow your cycle each day and ask yourself, "Am I fertile today?"

4. Remember that temperature can vary with travel, emotional changes or the time that you get up in the morning. Mark these changes on your graph and take them into account when figuring your safe and unsafe times.

BASAL TEMPERATURE RECORD

MONTH-YEAR

Day of Cycle	1	2	3	4	5	6	7	8	9	10	11	12	13	14	15	16	17	18	19	20	21	22	23	24	25	26	27	28	29	30	31	32	33	34	35
Day of Month																																			

99.0
.9
.8
.7
.6
.5
.4
.3
.2
.1
98.0
.9
.8
.7
.6
.5
.4
.3
.2
.1
97.0
.9
.8
.7
.6
.5
.4
.3
.2

BASAL TEMPERATURE RECORD

MONTH-YEAR

Day of Cycle	1	2	3	4	5	6	7	8	9	10	11	12	13	14	15	16	17	18	19	20	21	22	23	24	25	26	27	28	29	30	31	32	33	34	35
Day of Month																																			

```
99.0
  .9
  .8
  .7
  .6
  .5
  .4
  .3
  .2
  .1
98.0
  .9
  .8
  .7
  .6
  .5
  .4
  .3
  .2
  .1
97.0
  .9
  .8
  .7
  .6
  .5
  .4
  .3
  .2
```

BASAL TEMPERATURE RECORD

MONTH-YEAR																																		
Day of Cycle	1	2	3	4	5	6	7	8	9	10	11	12	13	14	15	16	17	18	19	20	21	22	23	24	25	26	27	28	29	30	31	32	33	34	35
Day of Month																																			

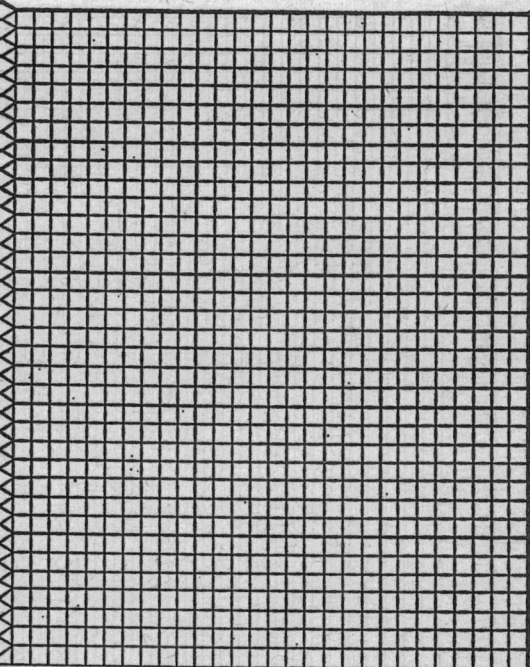

99.0
.9
.8
.7
.6
.5
.4
.3
.2
.1
98.0
.9
.8
.7
.6
.5
.4
.3
.2
.1
97.0
.9
.8
.7
.6
.5
.4
.3
.2

BASAL TEMPERATURE RECORD

MONTH-YEAR

Day of Cycle	1	2	3	4	5	6	7	8	9	10	11	12	13	14	15	16	17	18	19	20	21	22	23	24	25	26	27	28	29	30	31	32	33	34	35
Day of Month																																			

99.0
.9
.8
.7
.6
.5
.4
.3
.2
.1
98.0
.9
.8
.7
.6
.5
.4
.3
.2
.1
97.0
.9
.8
.7
.6
.5
.4
.3
.2

BASAL TEMPERATURE RECORD

MONTH-YEAR

Day of Cycle	1	2	3	4	5	6	7	8	9	10	11	12	13	14	15	16	17	18	19	20	21	22	23	24	25	26	27	28	29	30	31	32	33	34	35
Day of Month																																			

99.0
.9
.8
.7
.6
.5
.4
.3
.2
.1
98.0
.9
.8
.7
.6
.5
.4
.3
.2
.1
97.0
.9
.8
.7
.6
.5
.4
.3
.2

BASAL TEMPERATURE RECORD

MONTH-YEAR

Day of Cycle | 1 2 3 4 5 6 7 8 9 10 11 12 13 14 15 16 17 18 19 20 21 22 23 24 25 26 27 28 29 30 31 32 33 34 35
Day of Month

99.0
.9
.8
.7
.6
.5
.4
.3
.2
.1
98.0
.9
.8
.7
.6
.5
.4
.3
.2
.1
97.0
.9
.8
.7
.6
.5
.4
.3
.2

BASAL TEMPERATURE RECORD

MONTH–YEAR

Day of Cycle	1	2	3	4	5	6	7	8	9	10	11	12	13	14	15	16	17	18	19	20	21	22	23	24	25	26	27	28	29	30	31	32	33	34	35
Day of Month																																			

99.0
.9
.8
.7
.6
.5
.4
.3
.2
.1
98.0
.9
.8
.7
.6
.5
.4
.3
.2
.1
97.0
.9
.8
.7
.6
.5
.4
.3
.2

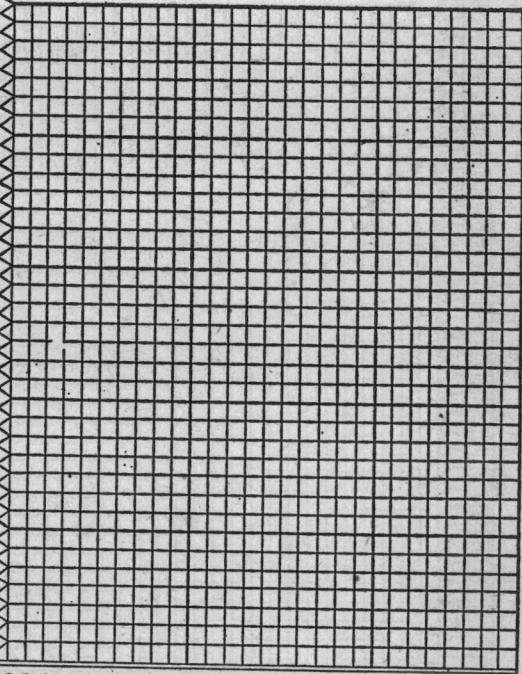

BASAL TEMPERATURE RECORD

MONTH-YEAR

Day of Cycle	1	2	3	4	5	6	7	8	9	10	11	12	13	14	15	16	17	18	19	20	21	22	23	24	25	26	27	28	29	30	31	32	33	34	35
Day of Month																																			

99.0
.9
.8
.7
.6
.5
.4
.3
.2
.1
98.0
.9
.8
.7
.6
.5
.4
.3
.2
.1
97.0
.9
.8
.7
.6
.5
.4
.3
.2

BASAL TEMPERATURE RECORD

MONTH-YEAR

Day of Cycle

Day of Month

BASAL TEMPERATURE RECORD

MONTH-YEAR

Day of Cycle	1	2	3	4	5	6	7	8	9	10	11	12	13	14	15	16	17	18	19	20	21	22	23	24	25	26	27	28	29	30	31	32	33	34	35
Day of Month																																			

99.0
.9
.8
.7
.6
.5
.4
.3
.2
.1
98.0
.9
.8
.7
.6
.5
.4
.3
.2
.1
97.0
.9
.8
.7
.6
.5
.4
.3
.2

BASAL TEMPERATURE RECORD

MONTH-YEAR																																		
Day of Cycle	1	2	3	4	5	6	7	8	9	10	11	12	13	14	15	16	17	18	19	20	21	22	23	24	25	26	27	28	29	30	31	32	33	34	35
Day of Month																																			

99.0
.9
.8
.7
.6
.5
.4
.3
.2
.1
98.0
.9
.8
.7
.6
.5
.4
.3
.2
.1
97.0
.9
.8
.7
.6
.5
.4
.3
.2

period you may notice that your vagina feels dry. Using that last tampon may be uncomfortable, and although you may want to make love you might find it hard because you feel dry. This absence of lubrication is characteristic of postmenstrual, low estrogen levels, of your body. As the estrogen level increases, your cervix produces a rich, slippery secretion which is an ideal medium for sperm to live in. This is the fertile mucus discussed in Chapter Four.

The other important hormone, progesterone, is released in large quantities afer the egg leaves the ovary. It functions to prepare the lining of the uterus to accept the fertilized egg, and is sometimes called the "baby saver." Without progesterone the fertilized egg would not be able to live and grow inside the uterus. Therefore, levels of progesterone are high during a pregnancy. If, however, an egg is not fertilized, progesterone levels will remain high for about two weeks and then drop off. The withdrawal or dropping off of the progesterone level corresponds with the beginning of the next period. While the progesterone level is elevated, your BBT will be elevated, too.

Progesterone comes from the ovarian follicle in much the same way that the estrogen does. After the release of the egg, estrogen production drops off in favor of progesterone. Progesterone production, on the other hand, increases and remains high until shortly before the next period. It is still produced from the follicle, which is now the place "where the egg used to be." Once the egg leaves, this area begins to break down. In the degenerative process, it turns yellow in color. This little bit of digression is important only so that you will remember the name of the progesterone producer—the corpus luteum, which means "yellow body" in Latin. Progesterone does not affect the secretions from your cervix, so it is the lowering of the estrogen rather than the increase in progesterone that changes the mucus at the end of your cycle.

The changes in BBT and mucus secretions discussed in Chapters Two through Four are related to hormonal fluctuations:

1. Estrogen, which increases as you move toward ovulation, causes the secretion of the wet, slippery, stretchy mucus, which, because it is hospitable to sperm, is called *fertile mucus*.

2. Progesterone, most of which is released after ovulation, causes the uterus lining to thicken, preparing it for the possibility of a fertilized egg. It also raises BBT.

3. When no fertilized egg attaches to the uterine wall, the amount of progesterone gradually decreases. This decrease causes the lining to be shed in the form of a menstrual period.

Demystification of Our Fertility Cycle

Understanding female anatomy and the changes your reproductive system goes through during each month's fertility cycle should bring you closer in touch with your body and create some positive feelings about yourself. An attractive part of this method of contraception is that you can follow your mood changes with your reproductive cycle. The same hormones that regulate your fertility also have a significant effect on your energy level, emotions, sexuality and sensuality.

Some women note that personality and energy variations correlate positively with hormonal changes throughout their cycle. These are not female "vapors" or "moodiness," but actual rhythmic changes that can be charted along with the fertility cycle. High energy has a definite pattern for some. Chris always finds that she exercises with most endurance four days before her period. Other women report that their sexual feelings change during their cycle. Women note "sensual" days, more inner-directed and cuddly, and "sexual" days, more outerdirected and actively sexual.

Do a survey on yourself by marking your moods, energy levels, feelings or whatever seems important on your graphs and correlate this information with temperature and mucus changes. You'll begin to understand how these necessary body regulators affect your body functions, your emotions, your energy level. This self-directed research is interesting and enlightening.

Review

1. Our bodies are rhythmical, logical and understandable.

2. The menstrual cycle is just that: a circle that repeats itself, with the end of one part flowing into the beginning of the next part.

3. Two hormones, estrogen and progesterone, affect fertility. The former changes the quality of mucus and the latter alters BBT after ovulation has occurred.

4. Energy levels, moods, sexuality/sensuality and other factors can be related to our menstrual cycle changes. We need to do self-directed research to define for ourselves what we feel at different times in the cycle.

CHAPTER SEVEN

Why Some People Fail at Birth Control

Now that you have learned how to use Natural Family Planning it is important to explore whether it is really for you. One way to do this is to look into why people fail at using contraception. All of us have a mixture of complex feelings in the area of sexuality, loving and birth control. Sometimes these feelings are angry, sometimes they are frightened and often they are very ambivalent. Any and all of these feelings are likely to conflict with the optimum use of Natural Family Planning, since this new contraception program requires a large degree of discipline and motivation. Thus, it is not surprising that most doctors shy away from advising this method for their patients. If they perceive their patients to have any conflicts about pregnancy and sexuality, they are probably justified in thinking that using Natural Family Planning is likely to result in unwanted, unplanned pregnancies.

It is striking that even fairly fool-proof methods of birth control like the pill and IUD have unwanted pregnancies associated with their use. This is because we are often in conflict about our use of contraception. It is not unheard of for a woman to forget to take a pill, or two, or three or even four pills in midcycle. This is usually more than just forgetting, just as forgetting to take one's diaphragm on vacation or on a date is more of a subconscious plan than an oversight. In short, no method is fool-proof if people are not going to be rational and disciplined.

Women are not the only ones to blame in this morass of contraceptive emotions. Men have so completely abrogated their responsibility for contraception that it is no wonder that women resent the carefree position of the male. The sex act is one in which two people participate and hopefully derive pleasure, yet it is generally the woman who has had to take the precautions. If we really think that sex is a manifestation of our loving, our caring, and our commitment to each other, then it is shameful that women should have to take all the responsibility for contraception. There is nothing admirable about a man who feels no responsibility for contraception merely because he is biologically not the one who gives birth to the baby. If women have sometimes been remiss in living up to the responsibility of birth control, men are just as much to blame for their almost complete lack of concern in this matter.

It is therefore doubtful that any single chemical method or device will solve all our problems in the area of contraception. Things won't be right until we work out our emotions in the areas of child bearing, sexual relationships and loving. Too many of our feelings influence our decisions in these matters for birth control to be only a medical and scientific problem. We believe that even if medical science came up with a safe, easy to use, and inexpensive birth control device there would still be unplanned pregnancies.

While there have been a multitude of articles and books written on the psychology of human sexuality, little has been written about the psychology of contraception methods. This chapter is a summary of this research to date, presented in the form of case studies. We are going to present *fictionalized* women who have had unplanned pregnancies or problems with contraception. The women are therefore contraception abusers. And so are the men who have participated in the problem, because just as a desired pregnancy requires a consenting man and woman, an unplanned pregnancy requires the carelessness of two people. Some of these cases represent abusers who are non-users—they have never used any method of birth control, even though they engage in sexual relations. Others represented in these fictionalized stories are just unhappy, alienated, or confused. The people are not real, but the feelings they have and the decisions they make are based on research data that was originally compiled from real people.

It is very probable that these stories will present situations with feelings and thoughts similar to those that you or your friends have had at one time. We hope that they will help you examine your own emotions, so that you may make an honest and intelligent appraisal of your use of Natural Family Planning.

Case 1: Mary is 26 years old and single. She has been going out with a number of different men since she broke up with her last steady boyfriend a year and a half ago. When she was with him she used a diaphragm. Now, she takes the birth control pill because it allows her to have spontaneous sexual relationships. She never has to interrupt love making with a man and put in her diaphragm, and she thinks that most men won't want to use a condom.

When she first started taking the pill a part of her thought that the pill would make her sexier, and help her have better sex. Since she didn't want to jump into a committed relationship right away, the pill seemed like the best way to avoid the discussion of birth control with each new boyfriend.

Oddly enough after taking the pill for a year she started to feel less inclined towards sexual relationships. Rather than feeling totally free about sexuality she has become a little depressed about it, and the pill seems to be a focus of this resentment. She doesn't really like taking a pill every day, now that she has sexual intercourse irregularly. It also seems to her that she is taking a precaution that may not be entirely good for her health, and she doesn't like the fact that men never seem to have to do anything that is harmful for their bodies.

Case 2: Bonnie is 32 years old and has been taking the pill for eight years. She has one child from a marriage that ended in divorce six years ago. Since then Bonnie has tried the IUD, but had it taken out after a year. During that time she had very heavy periods that often lasted two weeks. One time she had to go to a hospital emergency room because she had severe abdominal cramps. She was scared then that the IUD was giving her a serious infection, and after the episode was over had it removed. Since then she has taken the pill religiously.

She feels that she would take the pill even if there was a birth control method for men to use that was *foolproof*. Deep inside she is not sure that men would be reliable enough to take any birth control precaution regularly. She wants to have contraception completely in her own control. She even thinks that using contraception might make some men impotent because it disturbs their psyches.

Bonnie would actually like to find some way out of the dilemma, but the risks of not taking the pill and having another child alone seem too great. She does not want to have the responsibility of raising a child all by herself, and she is not sure that she can trust any man to share the responsibility for children.

Some of the important points of these two stories demonstrate the fact that women who feel insecure about their partners and their love relationships are also likely to feel this insecurity in the area of birth control. This becomes manifested in wanting complete control over birth control, and a lack of feeling that men want to share in the responsibility of family planning (which is all too often the case). Also, the fear of pregnancy can diminish a woman's desire to have sex, and once this desire falls off, having to use a method of birth control every day is likely to breed further resentment. Some of the reasons that women fear pregnancy are:

1. Having the financial burden of raising a child, especially if it means raising it alone.

2. Having a baby may be dangerous to one's health, especially if the woman feels that she is too old to be having one.

3. Having a baby is going to reduce one's sexual appeal.

4. Having the sole responsibility for raising a child is awesome.

5. The emotional trauma and possible physical side effects of having an abortion.

Given these feelings, it is no wonder that many women dive into using the most effective method of birth control, the pill, even if they are having sex on an irregular basis. Often the use of the pill may engender resentment, but the price of an unwanted pregnancy seems too dear to not take it. Moreover, many women feel that men regard the diaphragm or condom as "unsexy" and won't want to have a relationship with a woman who wants to use these methods.

Case 3: Barbara is 19 and has been going out with Bill for 3 years. They have been going steady since 11th grade, and she would very much like to get married. Right now they are both in their second year at the local community college. He wants to be an engineer, and she wants to be a teacher, although she is less sure of her plans than he is about his.

Barbara and Bill have been sleeping together since their senior year in high school. They didn't use contraception at all until her period was late for three weeks. When she realized what it would be like to have to tell her parents that she was pregnant, she immediately made an appointment at a birth control clinic and obtained oral contraceptives. Luckily, she wasn't pregnant, and was able to start on the pill with only an unpleasant emotional scare.

Last month Barbara lost her pocketbook with her pills in it, and didn't get a new prescription for about two weeks. During that time she still had sex with Bill. She didn't tell him that the pills were in her pocketbook, and he never thought to ask. They just continued to sleep together.

Somewhere inside of Barbara she probably wanted to get pregnant. Part of her felt that having a baby would cement her relationship with Bill a little more and make him want to get married. Also, she had been feeling more grown up than the other girls in her class, and having a baby seemed more mature than going to the community college.

Case 4: Jean is 21 and has been pregnant three times since she started having sexual relations at the age of 16. She's had one baby which she has been raising by herself, and two abortions. The first time she got pregnant she wasn't using any birth control at all. Her family had been very strict about sex, and had never talked about contraception while she was growing up. And as a teenager she had never been able to be open about wanting to have a boyfriend, much less sex, and had never considered preparing for it with contraception.

Shortly after she had the baby she moved out of her parents' home, and has not lived there since. She's done various things for a living, but has never stayed with one job very long.

Jean's second pregnancy was with a man that she was pretty serious about. She had been taking the pill, and somehow forgot to take a few pills in the middle of her cycle. She had intercourse anyway, thinking that she probably wouldn't get pregnant. When she did get pregnant, she and her boyfriend had a big fight about it. He didn't want a child, and she reluctantly got an abortion. Shortly after the abortion they had a really big fight and he moved out.

Her last pregnancy was a year ago. She hadn't had any relationships with men for a while after her last boyfriend moved out, so she wasn't using any contraception at all. One night she went to a party and slept with a man that she had never met before. She figured that she wouldn't get pregnant because she had just finished having her period. When she did find out that she was pregnant she immediately made arrangements for an abortion.

These two cases demonstrate how many women and men see having a baby together as a sign of a healthy and secure relationship. Often one party may want a baby as a sign that the other person really loves them and wants to stay forever. And for some having a baby may be a way to show one's family and friends that they are truly grown up. Thus, it is not surprising that a young person who is uncertain about her/his future may feel that having a baby is "the right thing to do."

Studies show that young people who use contraception early tend to have a higher level of ambition and a feeling that there is a rewarding future ahead. Much of this comes from the family. A family that encourages a child to succeed and reinforces the notion that there is a good future ahead is more likely to encourage a sensible attitude towards birth control and sex. Also, when a young woman feels alienated from the future—from the possibility of having a rewarding job, or a secure position in society—she is much more likely to feel hopeless about the use of birth control. Thus, if you feel out of control about your position in society, you are likely to feel that your reproductive functioning is also beyond your control. Conversely, if you feel that the present and future are likely to hold great success for you, you are much more likely to be concerned and fastidious about birth control.

Case 5: Judy and Ralph have been married for five years and have never had any children. This has been a constant source of tension between them. When they were first married Judy wanted to have children, but Ralph did not. He made her take the pill, and she resented it all the time. She felt that the pill was actually robbing her of her sexual drive and she rarely wanted to make love. When they did make love she didn't seem to get much pleasure out of it. Having sex when they weren't planning to have children seemed wrong somehow. She felt that it wasn't feminine and natural to be married and not planning to have children.

After almost two years on the pill she convinced him that having a child would be a good thing for both of them. She stopped taking the pill. However, she didn't become pregnant, and this caused a very real problem. Now he complains that she is barren and frigid, and she wants to have sex less and less. The more she rejects his advances, the more he seems to demand sex. She feels guilty about denying him sexual pleasure and gives in reluctantly, and only when she feels she has to to keep the marriage going.

Judy is a woman who feels that being married and having sex is justified only when procreation is planned. To her, contraception is an attack on her femininity. Many men also see a childless marriage as the fault of a "barren and frigid" woman. At one time it was hypothesized that the pill acted to lower a woman's sexual drive by the action of the hormones. If this is true it is only part of the problem. It seems that sexual satisfaction for many women, and potency for men, is often linked with childbearing. In childless marriages, contraception, or the inability to have children, often causes emotional problems that hinder sexual fulfillment.

Case 7: Margaret uses the diaphragm and hates it. She is married for the second time and has two children—one from her first marriage and one from her second marriage. Her marriage now seems to be going well and her life seems pretty stable. Sometimes she and her husband think about having another child, but they are uncertain about it, and put off the decision whenever it comes up.

Margaret has used every method of birth control on the market. As a teenager she had sex without using any contraception and was fortunate not to have had an unwanted pregnancy. By the time she was going out regularly with her first husband-to-be, she was on the pill. After the birth of her first child her gynecologist suggested that an IUD might work well, especially since she had already had a child. But, she didn't like the IUD because she feared having a foreign body inside her all the time.

She and her second husband have tried both the condom and diaphragm. For a while they alternated between the two methods, but now they rely upon the diaphragm most of the time. She wanted him to use the condom because she thought it would be fair for both to share in the birth control problem. But, neither of them really liked it. He hated it, and when she realized that he disliked it so much, she resigned herself to using the diaphragm all the time. Unfortunately she hates the diaphragm almost as much as he hated using the condom. Over all she feels that it is the safest method for her health, but she dislikes the mess and the lack of spontaneity.

Now they cheat on using the diaphragm whenever possible. She avoids using it for all but one week in the middle of her cycle. They are ambivalent about having another child. They figure that if Margaret gets pregnant they'll decide whether they want to have another child or go through with an abortion. However, they hope that they will be lucky and not have an unexpected pregnancy.

Margaret and her husband are caught in a common contraceptive dilemma. She considers every method to have drawbacks. The pill is dangerous to her health, the IUD frightening and the condom unsatisfying to her husband. There seems to be no ready solution, and "cheating" (not using the diaphragm some of the time) is a way of reducing the number of days when the problem must be encountered. However, both of them know that this cheating is risky and this too causes an undesirable tension.

The point of these case studies is that many people are ambivalent, confused, and dissociated from their sexuality and from the basic notion that intelligent family planning is part of mature sexuality. Many of us live in a hazy world of repressed feelings when it comes to sex. Few of us have either the Victorian values of sexual denial or the completely free feelings of so-called Aquarian liberation. We have one foot in the old world and one in the new, and our confused attitudes reflect this.

Moreover, the fact that all the available methods of contraception have drawbacks does not help our conflicting feelings. Some methods are potentially dangerous for our health, and some methods are ridiculously messy and inconvenient. And for some the whole concept of mechanical birth control runs against their ethical beliefs.

To review some of the points we have tried to make:

1. For many people it is hard to be completely guiltless about sexuality and pleasure. We still carry historical baggage that says that sex is dirty. In this light, it is no wonder that we repress our actions, and fail to take precautions in the form of birth control.

2. For some who find giving and receiving pleasure in a sexual relationship hard, it may be convenient to see sex only in terms of procreation. If enjoyment is lacking, having children makes the sex act meaningful.

3. We often express love in terms of having children. Men and women still feel that the hallmark of a good relationship is raising a child together. It is hard for some to relate for many years in a childless marriage without feeling that something is missing.

4. Even though we are living in an era when women seek fulfillment in careers and roles outside of the home and family, there is still a tremendous pull to equate femininity and maturity with childbearing and child raising. Even the most career-oriented woman feels at times that having and raising children is a good and positive part of being a woman. This conflict may make a woman feel ambivalent about years of sex with meticulous attention to contraception.

5. For some women having a child is seen as a form of giving.

6. If a woman feels depressed about her relationships with men, if she feels used, dependent, or angry, she is more likely to be irresponsible about contraception. Especially if other facets of her life, like being poor or stuck in a dull job with no future, reinforce this, she is likely to feel that she can't control her fertility. Having children or not having children may seem to be the work of chance or forces outside of her control, rather than her ability to control her own life.

7. There remains a basic inequality between the sexes where birth control is concerned. So far it has almost always been the sole burden of the woman.

How Women Feel About the Various Methods of Birth Control Available to Them

Approximately 4 out of 10 women who are having sexual relations have some fear of pregnancy. Some of the reasons that they fear pregnancy we have already stated. What is important is that they often see the burden of pregnancy and raising children as resting almost entirely on their shoulders. With all of these reasons it is no wonder that using a method of birth control becomes an important concern. Yet all the methods carry some drawbacks—either medical or psychological.

In a study where women were asked to pick an adjective from a list and associate it with a method of birth control, some very interesting results were obtained. First, women rarely felt that birth control was immoral or sinful. However, many of the available methods were described as unnatural, messy, unsafe or frightening.

Some of the interesting conclusions were:

1. 40% of the women polled felt that the pill was "unnatural."

2. Rhythm scored high on "femininity," "morality," good for "health" and low in "messiness." Considering that rhythm has had a bad name for its lack of reliability, these high scores are somewhat surprising. What these high scores seem to say is that women would like to find an alternative to the currently available methods of birth control, and would favor it if it were more reliable.

3. The condom was seen as unfeminine, unnatural, unsafe, repulsive, messy and unsatisfying.

4. The diaphragm scored low in the scale too, being seen as especially difficult, repulsive, messy and unfashionable.

5. Of all the methods, coitus interruptus scored the lowest most consistently.

We feel that this information indicates that if you are interested in Natural Family Planning you are not alone. When all the methods are considered together the pill is the least disliked, but rhythm is a close second. Actually, rhythm was considered to be more favorable on the scales for "femininity," and less likely to cause illness or be immoral. It was also rated as least unnatural, frightening or repulsive. Its major drawback is that it was considered unsafe. We believe that Natural Family Planning, when used properly, can eliminate this problem. We feel that for those who can adjust their sexuality to their natural fertility cycle this method is a viable alternative to the other available methods of contraception.

CHAPTER EIGHT

Emotional Reactions to Using the New Birth Control Program

In Chapter Seven we discussed many of the reasons why women and men abuse and misuse contraception. Natural Family Planning also has its abuses and the underlying reasons for these abuses. We know that the New Birth Control Program is very likely to fail if you have certain important psychological factors going against you. In this chapter we hope to outline for you many of these factors, so that you may be better able to decide if Natural Family Planning is right for you.

Even though you may be dissatisfied with your current method of contraception and concerned about the possible effects of the pill or IUD, you are very likely to have an unwanted pregnancy if you cannot adjust to the program. To use this program successfully, you must be satisfied with the routines that the method demands and be able to regulate your sexuality to your body cycles.

It is also critical that your male partner, whether he be your husband, lover or casual boyfriend, be able to adjust his sexuality to your body rhythms, and to accept that the method demands a new and unusual kind of communication about emotions, sexuality and abstinence.

Some Startling Facts

Here are some startling facts about the New Birth Control Program and human feelings based on a recent survey among couples using this method. Many of the facts are quite predictable and many are quite disturbing. We hope that as you read this chapter you can honestly apply these facts to your life to see if the method is workable for you. It is important to remember that of the many dangerous side effects of contraception, pregnancy is among the most dangerous. Any pregnancy carries potential medical risks, and an unwanted pregnancy carries the dangerous and lifetime problems of emotions for you, your mate and your children.

Most of the observations we will make in this chapter come from studies of the Catholic families using the method. While these families represent a selected sample, we believe that they still contain information relevant for all of us. These are observations that describe the interpersonal and sexual relationships of many adults, and for that reason are valuable to anyone interested in using the program.

How Men Dominate Women

1. In most sexual relationships the man was almost twice as likely to find the abstinence difficult, and he became more conscious of sex during the abstinence period.

2. If the man interpreted the charts the woman was more likely to get pregnant.

3. If the man found it difficult to abstain during the unsafe time, and the woman knew that he was unhappy about the abstinence, she was twice as likely to become pregnant.

These facts seem to point to the problem of male dominance in the sexual relationship. If the woman bows to the man's advances, even though she knows that she is possibly fertile, the method will not work.

Both men and women must take responsibility for pregnancy and its prevention, even though only one person carries the baby. In the conventional relationship the woman has often given in at her own expense. This attitude is particularly dangerous if you want to use Natural Family Planning.

We hope that the New Birth Control Program will promote added equality in the sexual relationship. Mutual responsibility in a relationship exists in sexuality, child rearing, household chores, and every other aspect of a good loving relationship. There is nothing unmasculine about a man and woman following a woman's fertility cycle in the sexual relationship.

There is also a limitless set of possibilities in a sexual relationship besides the male's ejaculation into the woman's vagina. Sexuality is loving, understanding, touching, being close, and exploring possibilities. Experience tells us that the method is not likely to work if the man cannot relate to abstinence, nonintercourse kinds of sex, and talking about the sexual relationship in general.

If you use a diaphragm and condom already, this merely means realizing when you need to use these devices and being honest about your fertility. You must also be aware that sexual intercourse with these devices during your fertile time carries a risk, although we believe it to be small if you use them properly. For couples who already use these devices the adjustment is easier than for couples in which the woman has always taken the pill or had an IUD. In any case, the method is not likely to work if the man and the woman are unable to communicate about sex and experiment with other kinds of sexuality beside male penetration.

Responses to Abstinence

1. Half of the couples who avoided sex *completely* during the unsafe times found that it had a negative effect on their relationship.

2. 45% of the men found the abstinence period dif-

ficult, while only 22% of the women found it difficult.

3. Two thirds of the couples felt that the abstinence period enhanced their appreciation of sex.

4. Women are more likely to worry about getting pregnant while learning the method. And almost half of them continued to worry about pregnancy even after practicing the method safely for a while. If you are concerned that these percentages do not add up to 100%, it is because they are responses to separate questions. Thus, the couples were considered as a unit, then the men separate from the women, and so on. We hope that these responses are understandable in the form they are presented. If you are interested in the study, see the *References Section* at the back for *Marshall and Rowe, 1970 and 1972*.

It is pretty clear that for most couples, men find it harder to adjust to sexual abstinence. We don't believe that women find sexual abstinence easier for biological reasons only. Enjoying sexuality for women has always been a problem when unwanted pregnancy is a possible result. It is not surprising that the woman, who has to carry the baby, and often bear the major burden of raising it, finds abstaining easier. This only seems to confirm the idea that the enjoyment of sexuality for women needs to be separated from childbearing when pregnancy is not desired.

Given that this pressure exists, it is not surprising that women worry more than men about getting pregnant while learning the method. Also, they are more likely to continue worrying even after using it successfully for a while. We believe that very few women of childbearing age ever lose their concern about pregnancy. If you are worried about pregnancy using this method you are definitely not alone. You should use this concern to your advantage by being extra cautious. You should be certain to avoid unprotected intercourse until you are certain that your fertile (unsafe) time has passed.

How men and women relate to the abstinence period

will determine, to a large extent the overall effectiveness of Natural Family Planning in preventing unwanted pregnancies. If the couple avoids all forms of love making during the unsafe time this is likely to cause a severe tension for the relationship. However, other forms of sexuality like mutual masturbation, oral sex, hugging and tenderness can make the abstinence time rewarding in its own right. It becomes a time of "just another kind of sexuality," as one couple has said. And, of course, for those people who normally use the diaphragm or condom the abstinence period is no different from their usual contraception routine. For those couples, the effort to pinpoint ovulation allows them to reduce the time that they already use these devices by a half to two thirds.

Social Factors

1. The older the husband and the older the couple the less likely they are to have an unplanned pregnancy.

2. The longer the couple is married, the less likely they are to have an unplanned pregnancy.

3. If the couple feels for economic and social reasons that their family size is exactly what they would like it to be, they are less likely to have an unplanned pregnancy.

4. In one study it was found that if both the partners were Roman Catholic they were less likely to have an unplanned pregnancy (as opposed to mixed marriages).

5. Socioeconomic factors seem to have no effect on the likelihood of having an unplanned pregnancy.

These facts tend to say that stability and reliability make the New Birth Control Program work. If you really feel that for financial and emotional reasons you cannot have another child you are likely to be very strongly motivated to follow the program faithfully. Also, if you have been together with your mate for a considerable amount of time and are older you prob-

ably have worked out your modes of communication
and your feelings a little better and are more likely to
be successful with the method.

We live in an age where free sexuality and liberation
are considered "hip." To be able to jump into bed with
a nameless, faceless member of the opposite sex at any
given time has been associated with "liberated" people. This kind of sexuality is difficult with Natural
Family Planning. It takes an element of control to tell a
new partner that you are ovulating and cannot have
sexual intercourse. It is hard to limit your new en-
counters to cuddling or sex without penetration in this
society where sexual intercourse is generally expected.
Thus, it is not surprising that older couples, more
stable couples, and couples with more time together are
less likely to have unplanned pregnancies using the
New Birth Control Program.

In summary, we are saying that motivation to make
the method work takes many forms. We have already
talked about the roles that family size, age, and stability
play in making the program work. It seems too that
religious and ethical beliefs play a part. Roman Catholic
couples clearly have a strong motivation to use the
method if they are already using Calendar Rhythm,
and feel that they cannot use any other birth control
method (or abortion) to control family size. In these
families, have an unwanted pregnancy, especially if
the family is already large enough to be an economic
burden, is a significant deterrent to careless behavior.
Natural Family Planning is the only method sanctioned
by the Roman Catholic Church, because it is natural.
Thus, couples who use this method (Natural Family
Planning) are really following the ethical principles of
their faith and have the added motivation of this con-
sciousness. And finally, it seems that income is not a
factor. What is important is that people come to Natural
Family Planning with a strong sense of personal motivation to make the method work. These people are the
most likely to be successful with it.

Teaching, Learning and Communicating

We know that the teaching quality and the length of time spent in teaching the method increases the success rate. While we believe that one can learn the method from a book, we also realize that it is more likely to be successful if it is learned in a group where questions and feelings can be discussed.

Unfortunately, in most places courses in Natural Family Planning are not available. Our own experience with a course in Natural Family Planning in our area involves four teaching sessions that run over four months. This allows women and men to chart at least four cycles under supervision, and to practice following the temperature and mucus methods before actually relying on them as methods of contraception.

In the first session the participants are given an introduction to the method of taking basal body temperatures, graphing and interpreting the BBTs, and a short lecture on the anatomy and physiology of human reproduction. They then go home for one month and begin to take their temperatures and follow their cycles. In the second session the mucus method is taught, and the women (men, too) go home for another month to follow these changes along with the temperature graph. During the third session the participants discuss their experiences and begin to put it all together.

This third session is an opportunity for people to discuss problems and feelings. Teaching the program is rather simple, but dealing with the emotional problems is much more difficult. We know that most of the failures have to do with human emotions rather than failures of the method itself. It is therefore not surprising that couples who learn the method in a group, where careful teaching and a forum where discussion of problems is available, do far better. Thus, the third session is an important time to discuss the problems that arise when one begins to use Natural Family Planning.

After the third session the couples go home and continue to chart temperatures and observe the mucus changes. The fourth session is a repeat of the third session plus a complete gynecological exam. By the fourth session each participant should have four months of charts to review and be able to point out the safe and unsafe times in the menstrual cycle. And of course, the fourth session is a time to discuss problems and feelings that arise in using the method. Thus, even though the couples are not actually using the method for contraception, they are beginning to learn what it means to their relationships to use the method. In this environment we believe couples will be better prepared to use the method and work out the problems that arise.

Self-Evaluation

1. If one member of the couple finds the method unsatisfactory they are about three times as likely to have an unplanned pregnancy.

If you are unhappy with this method of birth control and cannot work it out with yourself and your mate you should not be using the New Birth Control Program. The success of any method of contraception involves regular participation. In the case of the NBCP this is magnified greatly. If you are not happy about following your cycle every day and regulating your sexuality according to its natural rhythms you are likely to be sloppy and have an unplanned pregnancy. The problem is just about as severe if it is your mate who is unhappy with the program. Thus, if after a fair trial and discussion with your mate you or he are not satisfied, be fair with yourself and choose another method of contraception. You will be saving yourself the pain and anguish of an unwanted conception.

2. Conservative estimates say that one third to one half of all couples switch their method of contraception.

If you do not like the New Birth Control Program it is not the end of the world. Few men and women spend a lifetime with one method of contraception, and in fact many methods are available. We cannot think of anyone that we know who has relied upon the same method for an entire fertile lifetime. As you grow and change, your needs for contraception change. So may your feelings about Natural Family Planning.

Responsible Loving

We have tried to emphasize in this chapter the importance of responsible loving as the foundation for success of the New Birth Control Program. Attitudes about sexuality have changed so rapidly in the last generation that it all sometimes seems "too much too soon." If you think of the New Birth Control Program as a way to control fertility by periodic abstinence you are most likely to succeed. It is a method of contraception only if both female and male can regulate their sexuality to the woman's fertility cycle.

Taking responsibility for one's sexuality involves knowing what you want from a close relationship. The problems that arise from using the program are those that involve interpersonal communication, mutual effort, a sense of knowing what you want, and an element of self-control. Women must ask themselves if *"giving in"* is right, and men must question whether *demanding* selfish pleasure is fair. We do not want to imply that single women should not use the method, but that everyone must be able to decide for themselves what they want from their sexual relationships and be honest about the obvious reality that pregnancy is a possible consequence of making love. It is not hard to be successful with the New Birth Control Program. We have been using it and find it very rewarding. But it does take a desire to maintain responsible loving.

Review

1. Studies show that both men and women find the abstinence period difficult. Although it is disliked more by men than by women, the success of the program depends on how both people in the re-

lationship relate to the demands of periodic abstinence.

2. Finding ways of loving without male penetration
   can make the abstinence period less of a problem.

3. Social factors such as family size, the compatibility
   of the partners, and age seem to play a role in the
   success of the program.

4. We believe that responsible loving means communicating needs and maintaining openness in the relationship. Men and women who can talk about
   their sexual needs and feelings are more likely to be
   successful with the New Birth Control Program.

CHAPTER NINE

Variations, History and Future Trends

This is a chapter of additions. It covers some subjects that people have asked us to include but that did not seem to fit in any previous part of the book. The first section covers the relationship of basal body temperature to temperature taken at other times in the day. It shows that there is a relationship between your body metabolism, temperature and time of the day, and that it all correlates with your morning basal reading. We do not advise regular use of temperatures from diverse times for following your fertility cycle, but this can be used on occasion when you forget to take your morning temperature.

The next three sections deal with special kinds of temperature graphs. The first, "Temperature Cycles that Never Go Up," is a caution not to consider every monophasic temperature cycle as anovulatory. In many cases women may have a month in which there is no sustained rise, but they have in fact ovulated. The next part deals with the effects of drugs on your temperature. The information presented in this section deals with the pharmacological properties of the drugs, rather than controlled studies using these drugs and recording BBTs. This is because such studies have yet to be done. It is important for anyone using drugs and Natural Family Planning to realize that these agents can alter your temperature chart. And finally, we consider the effect of certain disease states on temperature.

The last part of the chapter deals with the history of Natural Family Planning and some view to the future. We believe that further investigation into the female fertility cycle will give us new and better ways to follow ovulation and to use this knowledge as a method of birth control.

What If You Forget to Take Your Morning BBT?

Everyone forgets to take their basal body temperature once in a while. Sometimes you are too busy, sometimes you remember later in the day, and sometimes you forget entirely. If you get up, and haven't taken your temperature there is a way to convert a nonbasal reading into a fairly accurate basal one. Here is the formula:

$$5 \text{ p.m. Temperature} - 0.7°F \ ^5 \ BBT \ (Approximate)$$
$$\text{BEDTIME Temperature} - 0.3°F = BBT$$

This formula was developed by researchers who had women record their morning BBTs, 5 p.m. and bedtime temperatures. When these three readings were graphed the picture showed that the three curves were very similar. The afternoon (5 p.m.) temperature was the highest, the morning temperature was the lowest, and the bedtime temperature was in between. What is most important is that when the temperature rose, signaling that ovulation has passed for the basal body temperature readings, it also rose for the other readings. If you remember that your temperature is a measure of your body's metabolism, and that sex hormones affect your metabolism, it is not surprising that they would affect it all through the day.

We do not recommend using this conversion very often, and we suggest that you try to take a morning, evening and bedtime reading of your own to see how your own body operates. The conversion numbers that we have given above represent an average. It may not be exact for you, and you would not want to have an unplanned pregnancy just because you are not "average." What is important is that there is a relationship among morning, afternoon and evening metabolism that is relatively fixed. And, this relationship can be used to help you keep track of your cycle if you forget to take your morning reading.

When you use a non-BBT temperature, mark it on your chart as a reading from a different time of day (See "The Importance of Establishing Your Daily Routine," page 22). You will become familiar with your charts after a few cycles and will be able to evaluate your non-BBT readings to see if they make sense. If you do not mark these readings correctly your graph will be difficult to interpret. Above all, be cautious about using these readings if you are uncertain about your ovulation. Overall we are looking for a biphasic curve. You should be able to see this curve even in the presence of a temperature taken at a non-BBT time. When in doubt be sure to check your temperature observations with your mucus and anatomy as we have described earlier.

Temperature Cycles that Never Go Up
Sometimes the time of ovulation is hidden in cycles that appear to be monophasic. In other words, just because your temperature doesn't show a characteristic biphasic curve, with a sustained rise, it does not mean that you are necessarily having an anovulatory (no ovulation) cycle.

These readings don't alter the reliability of the New Birth Control Program but present some problems in terms of abstinence. If your temperature does not show a postovulatory rise, you are safe to have unprotected intercourse. In these cycles your abstinence period will continue throughout the month. However, as long as you obey the rule that you avoid unprotected intercourse until your temperature rises, you will not risk an unplanned pregnancy during that cycle. If you use the mucus method, your mucus symptoms will help tell you if you are in fact having an anovulatory cycle, and this should help cut down on the necessary number of days of abstinence for these cycles.

The occurrence of this phenomenon—monophasic (no rise) charts—is purely individual. Rarely will it happen more than once or twice in a year. What is essential is that you maintain abstinence from unprotected intercourse until you are certain that ovulation has in fact occurred for that month.

Drugs and Temperature

Many women are concerned about the number of factors and agents that can alter their basal body temperature. Certainly, this method would not be reliable if every small change in your body made your BBT inaccurate. Some drugs, however, do change your body temperature, and you should be careful to note on your chart if you have been taking drugs.

For instance, barbiturates like Seconal[T] and Nembutal[T] lower metabolic rate and therefore lower your temperature if taken in sufficient quantities. This is also true of Valium[T], although it is less known for its metabolic depression than barbiturates. Phenothiazenes, which are strong tranquilizers (e.g. Thorazene[T], Compazene[T]), can elevate your temperature. Morphine, heroin, and codeine are strong narcotics that can lower your temperature if taken in sufficient amounts.

Stimulants speed up your metabolism. Thus, high doses of cocaine can elevate your temperature by stimulating your system. So can amphetamines. And alcohol, our most common intoxicant, can either stimulate or depress your system depending on the amount you take. No temperature studies on marijuana are available to our knowledge.

If you note on your temperature chart that you had been to a party and been drinking the night before, you will see over a period of time the effect of drinking on your temperature. Similarly, if you note the use of

Valium^T or Seconal^T on your temperature chart you will begin to have a good reference for your own body actions. Being a good investigator merely means being accurate and faithful in noting changes. Some women say that drinking the night before raises their morning BBT, others say that it seems to have little or no effect.

In general, stimulants will raise your temperature and depressants will lower it. Some drugs, like aspirin, have little effect on normal temperatures, but will effect an abnormal (elevated) one. The exact effect of drugs on BBT is hard to establish since drugs often effect different people differently, and there are many variables depending on the time you take them and the quantity you take. See for yourself. Be suspicious of temperatures that seem out of line with your normal cycle if you know that you have been taking drugs, been unusually anxious, or had less than your usual amount of rest.

Diabetes, Thyroid Disease, Obesity and Other Diseases
Many medical problems can cause amenorrhea (failure to menstruate) and/or infertility. Women with these conditions may also have a monophasic (no rise) basal body temperature chart. As a regular part of the medical investigation of a woman's fertility, many medical tests, including a basal body temperature chart, are performed. Conditions such as diabetes, thyroid disease, tumors of the adrenals, brain tumors, ovarian cysts and a host of other problems can all cause disruption of the normal menstrual cycle. In addition, anxiety and anorexia (not eating) can also cause changes in the normal menstrual cycle. While not all the disruptions of the menstrual cycle are due to serious disease processes, the failure to menstruate, prolonged period with a monophasic BBT chart or prolonged infertility should be investigated.

If you have a monophasic basal body temperature chart for one or two cycles per year, this is a normal condition. If you persist in having monophasic charts you should see a doctor and have this investigated. This is especially true if you have been feeling ill in association with the change in your periods. It is beyond the scope of this book to discuss the many factors that can cause a woman to fail to ovulate. Some of these problems are very serious, but on occasion failure to ovulate may be due only to stress. And, in most cases a full medical investigation into failure to ovulate and menstruate fails to uncover a medical reason for the problems. However, we do advise looking into this problem if you note a failure to have a normal biphasic curve for many months, a change in your periods, or a change in your cervical mucus.

The Past and the Future

The history of Natural Family Planning is a long one, at least as far as scientific ideas are concerned. Scientists have thought that a woman's menstrual cycle has a fertility pattern since at least the nineteenth century. This is not surprising since the bleeding of dogs and the "heat" pattern of other mammals has been recognized as a sign of fertility since the beginnings of animal husbandry. However, the nature of the cycle in women, and the role of temperature and mucus is a much newer idea.

In 1873, LeComte, a Belgian theologian, attempted to formulate a safe period for Catholic families who wanted to control family size without committing sin. Actually, the Church forced him to withdraw his writings and discontinue his investigations. However, it became necessary to reintroduce this idea after the introduction of the pessary (a cup designed to occlude the cervix) as a method of birth control in 1881. At that time the Church advocated the use of the Capellman Schedule, which considered the safe time to be between Day 14 and Day 25 of the menstrual cycle. Unfortunately, this was not very successful in preventing pregnancy since Day 14 was very likely to be the day of ovulation.

In 1924, a Japanese researcher named Ogino published a more scientific paper on the safe period. He understood that ovulation generally occurs in midcycle, and by 1932 had refined his work to a formula that considered a woman to be fertile from 12 to 19 days before her next menstrual period. Around the same time an Austrian named Knaus independently published work on the safe period. He maintained that the safe period was always 15 days before the next menstrual period.

Obviously, no researcher could predict when the next period would come, so a more generalized formula had to be developed. A composite formula that took into account the length of the woman's cycles was developed. Researchers disagreed somewhat on the exact formula and many formulas with slight differences were offered. The following is a simplified version of the Ogino-Knaus concept:

First day of fertile time =
    10 + # days in shortest cycle — 28
Last day of fertile time =
    17 + # days in longest cycle — 28

Thus, if a year had cycles that ranged from 26 days to 31 days in length, the formula would be computed as follows:

$$\text{First day of fertile time} = 10 + 26 - 28$$
$$= 8$$
$$\text{Last day of fertile time} = 17 + 31 - 28$$
$$= 20$$

Therefore this woman would not be safe from Day 8 through Day 20 of her cycle for every cycle in the year. Thus, she would have 13 days of abstinence each month.

As far as we are concerned this is all useless, other than for historical purposes. While this may work for most cycles, there is enough variation even within one woman's fertile life to make this method likely to result in an unplanned pregnancy. In addition, it lengthens the period of necessary abstinence, whereas the New Birth Control Program, which treats each cycle individually, provides one with many more safe days. In short, the Ogino-Knaus method attempts to predict ovulation on the basis of statistics. However, there is no way to predict ovulation. Only by following the anatomical and physiological changes that accompany the menstrual cycle each month can the approximate time of ovulation be determined.

The temperature method also has an interesting history. In 1905, Van de Velde noticed that the temperature of one of his patients dropped in the middle of her cycle and then rose to a plateau and was maintained at that level just prior to the day of menstruation. However, it wasn't until almost 30 years later that scientists began to understand the significance of this variation. In 1935, a German priest, Wilhelm Hillebrand, read Van de Velde's earlier work and decided to try an experiment with twenty women in his parish. He plotted the temperatures of these women and found the characteristic fall and rise associated with ovulation that is called the biphasic curve. What these researchers did not know at the time was that these temperature changes were due to changes in female sex hormones. As the endocrinology of the female system was explored, the significance of the temperature change was understood.

We are still in an early stage of scientific awareness in regard to following the female fertility cycle. The nature of the cyclic pattern is understood, but there is only a sketchy understanding of all the factors involved. As we learn more about the physiology of the female fertility system we will begin to find new and better tests for following the menstrual cycle.

The importance of the New Birth Control Program's use in family planning is that it uses simple inexpensive test(s) that can be used at home to follow the changes in a woman's fertility. Although this method works for many women, it is clearly not as easy as a test tape, tablet, or sign that could be used each day to tell when ovulation is about to occur. The problem is not only finding a simple test for determining the onset of ovulation, but one that would be sensitive at least five days prior to the event because sperm can live in the female tract for five days. Thus, if you ovulate on Day 15, your test tape must tell you to abstain from unprotected intercourse on Day 10.

It is not an impossible task. We know that the female body goes through a process of preparation before ovulation actually occurs. In fact, the female system is in a dynamic cycle that *culminates* in ovulation. Thus, we need a way to follow the regular cycle of changes that *lead to* the formation of the mature egg. Research in this area is being done all over the world by such groups as the World Health Organization, population control centers and individual scientists.

Some new ideas are:

1. A test for urinary estrogens, leutinizing hormones or other hormones that change during the cycle. The breakdown products of these hormones are in the urine, and a simple test for these substances is promising. However, the tape must be sensitive to small changes and be calibrated so as to warn of ovulation at least five days in advance.

2. Salivary tests. Changes in body estrogen also affect other enzymes like alkaline phosphatase, B-glucuronidase, and arylsulphatase. Exfoliation (sloughing) of cells also occurs in response to estrogen. This process can be seen in cells in the vagina and in the cheek.

3. Standardization of spinnbarkeit and ferning has been attempted, but the success has been very limited. We do know that the pattern of mucus with regard to stretchiness and cross linking changes with impending ovulation, but methods to standardize these phenomena have been unsuccessful. It would take a very experi-

enced person to be able to stretch her mucus and measure it exactly the same way each month, without a gage or meter.

4. Chloride testing has been available for some time, but it has not caught on as an ovulation detection method. We know that both chloride and potassium increase with ovulation and a test tape for the former has been tried. However, most women do not seem to favor this, and instead rely on the visualization of spinnbarkeit, and mucus quantity and quality. The test is also very sensitive to household cleaning agents. Thus, if a woman were to clean the insertion tube for the test tape in a sink that had been cleaned with a chlorine cleanser, the results would be inaccurate.

5. PH is a measure of the acidity or alkalinity of a medium. We know that the pH of the vagina is normally acidic and the mucus is basic (alkaline). This property of the mucus allows for sperm life. A simple pH test strip is available, but is often inaccurate due to variation in the overall pH of the vagina.

We are confident that as the work towards ovulation detection proceeds, better methods for following the menstrual cycle will be discovered and marketed. We welcome this as a medically safe way to control family size and for the promotion of the health and welfare of the society as a whole.

Review

1. You can use a non-BBT reading to keep your graph up-to-date for times when you forget to take your morning temperature. This method is less accurate, but can be used on occasion. In general, you should expect your afternoon temperature to be about 0.7°F higher than your morning reading, and your bedtime temperature to be about 0.3°F higher than your morning temperature.

2. Not all monophasic temperature charts indicate an anovulatory cycle. Don't have unprotected inter-

course just because you think that you are having an anovulatory cycle.

3. Certain diseases can affect ovulation, menstruation, and your basal body temperature. If you have pro-longed periods of a monophasic graph, or a failure to menstruate, you should see a physician, as this may be a signal of an ongoing disease process.

4. Certain drugs can also affect your temperature. If you are taking drugs you should note their use on your chart and interpret your graph assuming that these agents may have altered your basal body tem-perature.

CHAPTER TEN

Personal Accounts

The interviews on the pages that follow are stories of
people who are using the New Birth Control Program.
We have found their thoughts and feelings to be most
interesting, both in terms of their diversity and their
similarity. All those whom we have interviewed seem
to want an alternative method of birth control that is
in agreement with their ethical or religious beliefs, that
is medically safe and that allows them to enjoy a
mutually satisfying sexual relationship.

We hope that you enjoy these interviews and that
they shed some light on how the program is used—in
short, how this method of birth control can become
integrated into one's daily life.

John and Pat

Pat lives with her husband, John and their twins, a boy
and a girl aged 8, in a suburban area of upstate New
York. Pat, who is 29, works as an office manager for
an area legal firm. John, 27, is a psychiatric social
worker. They both enjoy living in the relatively open
spaces of upstate New York after growing up in New
York City.

Pat says their favorite family hobby is "hockey
watching." She explains that they have gotten into
supporting local hockey teams after her son started
playing the sport. In addition, both children are in
Little League and on wrestling teams (Pat says her

daughter is the only girl on the wrestling team, but is doing "really well.") Chris conducted the interview with Pat on a Saturday before the Christmas holidays. Pat likes to bake "all kinds of different foods," and was, this particular Saturday, making an amazing sausage and cheese stuffed bread that is a holiday favorite with her family. "It's sort of like pizza without the tomato sauce," she says. Pat and John have used the New Birth Control Program for a year now. "At first it seemed like every time I looked at her she had a thermometer sticking out of her mouth," jokes John, "but basically, I like it."

PAT: I was raised as a Catholic, but my mother didn't use rhythm. No one in my family seemed to use it, and I think that most Catholics don't practice it. I was taught in school and in Church that birth control was wrong, but I never really thought that Calendar Rhythm worked, so I didn't use it.

I've also known about the methods used in the NBCP for a long time. I guess that I always associated it with Calendar Rhythm, so I thought it was unreliable. Like many women, I have tried lots of different methods of contraception. At first I used a condom. Then, after the birth of my twins, I started taking the pill. After a while I went back to the condom, and then back to the pill for 2½ or three years. I stopped taking the pill because I developed cysts in my breasts. Also, during my cycle on the pill, my breasts would swell up and get so sore that I knew it was time to get off.

I've been to three doctors about these cysts and all have told me that there is nothing that can be done about them. They've told me to cut down on the salt, take vitamin B complex, and another doctor gave me a prescription that I never filled. I couldn't see spending a lot of money to get a prescription filled for something that might not work. At any rate, I haven't taken the pill since.

I've used a diaphragm for two years now, and I hate it. I've hated it since the day I got it. I hate it during the winter time, when living up here in Siberia like we do, I have to get out of bed when it is 20 degrees below zero. Then I have to put cold jelly in a cold diaphragm and put that in a warm me. By the time I get back into bed I am so cold that I am no longer interested in making love.

My husband likes this method too. He's somewhat skeptical about it as a birth control method, but he thinks that it's really neat to know your own body. He's thinking about taking his own temperature to see if he has a cycle. He thinks in part that by the time you're sure that you've ovulated it is so late that he's only getting a couple of days out of it. I don't mind that so much. We still use the diaphragm, and when we think that I am ovulating we don't have genital sex. That's new since we've been using the method. I've been much more conscious not to take any foolish chances since I have been taking my temperature.

I grew up with the attitude that you stay away from your body. There seemed to be no curiosity about it, certainly no satisfying curiosity about it. I think that it's a gas to know this about my body after so many years. You know that you go to gynecologists for years and ask questions and don't understand what they are talking about. I have always felt that if I keep questioning he's going to think that I am a jerk. Apparently, I am supposed to understand what he is telling me, but I often don't. The method has definitely increased my awareness of my own body.

I think that this will help me teach my daughter about menstruation. I now think that I have a very good attitude towards things. The other day my daughter came in while I was taking my temperature. She asked about it and I told her that it was something that I did everyday for my health. I think that as she grows up I won't have any trouble telling her about menstruation.

Bonnie and Steve

We interviewed Bonnie and Steve in their suburban upstate New York home on a very cold January day. Bonnie, who raises house plants as a hobby, says she first got into plants when she realized how little green she saw in their northern climate. Their four children, ranging in ages from 3 years to 10 years, wandered in and out during the interview.

Steve and Bonnie, who have been married for 11 years, have known each other since childhood. "I actually did marry the boy next door!", Bonnie says. Steve, who is 33, works as a real estate appraiser for the state government. At 32, Bonnie has been a Registered Nurse for 12 years. She has spent the last five years teaching the Lamaze childbirth method. She is also active in LaLeche League, an organization that promotes breast-feeding. She has breast-fed all of their children. "Some people think I'm a fanatic," she says, "but, I really believe it's best."

This "natural" way of doing things extends to many parts of their lives. They always have a big garden in the summer and can their homegrown vegetables for the winter months. These activities, and chopping wood for the fireplace, are done in part because they enjoy them and partly to help cut corners financially.

For vacations, Steve and Bonnie prefer to take the family camping for extended weekends. It's economical ("Feeding our crew at MacDonalds would cost $10.00!") and provides a time for real family interaction while appreciating the out-of-doors. Bonnie and Steve have been using the mucus observation alone as their family planning method for over three years. They had to rely on mucus while Bonnie was breast-feeding and found it effective enough for them. They have chosen to use it exclusively to prevent an unplanned pregnancy.

BONNIE: We've been using the mucus method for three years now. I knew about it before that, but never tried it. We began when our fourth child, Molly, was one month old, and as a matter of fact, we brought her to the first class. We felt that we had had our children and that our family was complete. Having four children, spaced pretty close together, seemed like enough.

I was raised a Catholic and I think that we started our married life with feelings about contraception from our religious backgrounds. We started with rhythm and basically didn't care when our first child came. We used to call it Aunt Jane's rhythm as a cute little joke. We even wondered after the first six months of being married why we didn't have a child on the way. So at first we didn't worry about contraception, but that is different now and we have really thought it through.

STEVE: I feel safe using the method because I trust Bonnie. She seems to be able to read her signs and know when the time is safe. It was a while before I felt completely confident using the method. Maybe it was because Bonnie was breast-feeding, but I think that it takes a while before you get to really know the signs. She felt that she was wet all the time at first, but what she learned was to distinguish the changes in the secretions. It was a fallacy that has come to pass that breast-feeding would keep her from ovulating. In fact she ovulated two months after having Molly. We actually used the temperature method for a few months to support the mucus method. I guess that it was really six months before we became confident that the method worked.

BONNIE: My biggest problem with contraception is that I have always breast-fed for a good length of time. The pill goes into your breast milk and I didn't want it to affect my offspring. So, the pill was out, and morally I wasn't interested in the IUD. You know, an IUD doesn't prevent conception; it only prevents pregnancy. What happens is that a fertilized ovum makes its way into the uterus and you abort it. We've never used a diaphragm or condom because of the lack of spontaneity, and the feeling of artificiality. We actually used Calendar Rhythm fairly successfully, but this is much more accurate.

Beginning the method is a little hard, because you feel pretty insecure. We started using both the temperature and mucus together, but with breaking thermometers and getting up with a small child we found the temperature method not to be useful. I even had doubts about the secretions while breast-feeding. It seemed to me that I was always wet even though they were talking about dry days. I now know that the main reason that it was so difficult for the first month was that I hadn't really started a cycle. We didn't know what the secretions meant because we didn't know where I was in my cycle. Surprisingly, the first cycle started with ovulation rather than menstruation because I was breast-feeding.

After my periods resumed I began to feel a little more confident. As it turns out the reason why I felt that I was wet during the first weeks of learning the method (and breast-feeding) was that I was getting ready to ovulate. I didn't know it then because we were so new to the method. I had never been aware of it before, but I had all the symptoms, like the slipperiness and the egg white secretion.

That was three years ago. We have stayed on the method ever since, even with Molly nursing for a long time. We got rid of the thermometer right away. When we were learning we thought that the thermometer was to reassure you about the secretions. When in doubt they said go with the secretions. I check my secretions by sensation generally and not necessarily feeling for it. If I am in doubt I check to see if it is stringy. Those times, like when I get a very wet sensation, I actually go into the bathroom and check it.

STEVE: Bonnie has said that I am a prime motivator in this method. I hadn't really thought of it that way. Right now we don't have any other method of contraception, or actually any other likeable method. I feel that I can live with this method. It is encumbent on both of us to use the method properly. I would find it hard to blame her if she got pregnant. So by me participating in it, the burden is on me, too. Maybe that makes it more acceptable too. It's not a selfish type thing where you say, "you take the pill," or "if you get pregnant it is your fault." This way the burden is shared by both of us.

We never cheat. I assume that the method is not foolproof. No method is. So when you cheat you have two things against you. We didn't cheat on Calendar Rhythm and Molly was conceived. We've had a few close calls and we know how it would feel to have an unplanned pregnancy. Maybe it's a selfish thing, but we do have four children and to have a fifth would mean more furniture, more beds, more clothes, the whole bit. There's enough in the back of my mind to prohibit me from cheating. It's a combination of common sense and fear.

BONNIE: Abstinence is the lesser of two evils. We feel that it is right to keep to the natural. I am a full-time mother, but I do other things. When people ask what I do, I say that I am a full-time mother and a part-time nurse. Molly was a Lamaze birth, completely unmedicated, and Steve was in the delivery room. We're both into Natural Childbirth, Natural Family Planning and LaLeche. So, abstinence is the lesser of the two evils.

We found that with a large family it wasn't always feasible anyway. So, you definitely have to arrange your [sexual] moods around your cycle. And I think that it's a lot in your mind. Steve always knows when I am ovulating without my telling him. He says that he can smell a difference. We have a red light-green light system that is kind of funny. You know, if I have the drawer open and the pajamas out it means one thing, and if I don't it means another. It's not the quantity of sex, but the quality. If you had candy all the time, and it was just sitting on the table you wouldn't want it so much anymore. I don't think that everyone agrees with me on that but Steve does, I know. And that's what is important. I have to emphasize that it has to be a two way street. This is one method that you can't do alone. If the abstinence is too much of a hardship for one or the other then it won't work.

With my cycle we have about 10 days of abstinence out of a 32 day cycle. When I tell other people about the method they are often skeptical. They think, why bother? But, you know, after a while it's not much of an effort. I would say that the hardest part for me is the abstinence, not finding out how my system works and following it. That's a neat thing. I make my chart for a few days at a time and keep it in the bedroom drawer. I am very accurate from when my period ceases until when I ovulate. I still keep track after that, but it is more relaxed. So, although the abstinence period is sometimes untimely, not every month is by any means a hardship. Vacations, believe it or not, we plan around my cycle.

STEVE: This is a topic of conversation among a lot of our friends. Some think that we are playing with fire, but they don't have any single method that they find satisfactory, either. We've talked about permanent methods like tubal ligation and vasectomy, but we haven't come up with a firm answer about it.

BONNIE: We had a scare in the fall. I woke up with a terrible pain in my side . . . like ovulation, but it was a week late. And then my period came a week and a half late that month. During the scare we began consoling each other that it wouldn't be so bad to have another child. When we have a scare it makes us feel more inclined towards sterilization. Neither of us really wants to do it, and we respect the right of the other person not to want to have it done to them.

STEVE: There is a question of how the future will go. I am 33 and Bonnie is 32. We've been using the method for three years but we still have many fertile years left. Do we really want to use this method and have the tension of possibly having unplanned pregnancies?

BONNIE: We still feel secure enough to stay with the method, but one failure might make us change our minds. But, I guess this applies to any method of birth control. There is an element of failure, even human failure, in all of them. For us it is still a question of the lesser of all evils. We've thought about all the forms, and this is the most likeable at this point in our lives.

I have already started to teach my ten-year-old about secretions and the cycle. Her secretions are beginning to change premenstrually, and in the last month I have begun to see that her secretions are getting heavier. I've talked about it with my pediatrician. I haven't talked about fertile versus non-fertile yet, but she knows that they will change from red to brown and go back to the color that she is used to seeing. When she actually starts her cycle I will definitely talk to her about how it changes. I don't know exactly what my motive is now, but it is nice for her to know what her body is doing.

Julie and Rob

Julie and Rob are both scientists. She works in a human reproduction laboratory and he is a plant biologist. They met in California, and have since moved to Brighton, Mass. She is 24 and he is 35. They don't have children now, but consider it as a possibility for the future.

They are very much involved with the New Birth Control Program and have researched it themselves, so that they feel very comfortable with it. Julie has never considered using the pill or IUD and has become more and more convinced that it is dangerous to interfere with the natural reproductive cycle of women. Rob is also very much interested in biorhythms, and is considering taking his own temperature and seeing how it varies with Julie's.

JULIE: I heard about the program from my sister who was taking a course in this method. I had always suspected that it was biologically possible to pinpoint the time of ovulation. I thought that if you could just figure out when you were ovulating you could have to use birth control for only a small part of the menstrual cycle.

I was a biology major in college and am currently working at the Human Reproduction Lab. In my work I have been exposed to projects that explore methods for pinpointing ovulation. Usually though, people use these methods to conceive rather than for contraception.

I have never used any of the chemicals or devices for birth control, and I certainly never considered taking the pill. Anybody who knows anything about reproduction, knows that the female has a rhythmic cycle that goes through changes on the hormone level. It just seems crazy to me to take a pill that disrupts this natural cycle.

ROB: I'm involved in this too. I'm a biochemist so this is interesting for me. I am generally aware of where she is in her cycle.

JULIE: When I began taking my temperature I had already been convinced that my cycle was very irregular. My cycle still varies in length, but it feels more regular because I can see its changes. I took my temperature for two months before using it as a method of contraception. During that time I did some reading in textbooks that verified the scientific basis of the method.

My reading convinced me that once the temperature rises, once there is a dip and rise, you are not going to ovulate again that cycle. So, when I observe the biphasic curve I am sure that ovulation has occurred and that I am safe.

In scientific research, every day you get data, information, and you analyze it. You look at that graph [pointing to her temperature chart], that data, and you interpret what you see. If you see weird things going on, you know that something weird is going on with you that month. Then you have to use alternate contraception for that time. On the other hand, if the graph is clear cut, if the temperature rose, and you have no reason to suspect you have a fever or anything, you can feel pretty confident. I know I do.

You don't have to be scientifically oriented to use the method. Of course, it's understanding the data. When you are a scientist doing a project you can interpret the information because you understand the process and then you can interpret the data. Once anyone understands about the biphasic curve, interpreting the temperature charts is pretty easy.

The lab I work in explores the area of human reproduction. There are a lot of people who work on temperature interpretation. Unfortunately, in their own lives they equate the use of temperature observation with Calendar Rhythm—they don't make the distinction. So, I was hesitant to tell people. I did finally tell the fellow I work with. As it turns out he and his girlfriend have decided to use condoms as the only safe method. He was a little taken aback that I was using temperature graphs, but he did agree with my feeling that the method is scientifically sound. He also felt that it was a workable method for some people. He also said that there were some people in the lab working on ways to pinpoint ovulation by testing for certain substances that are secreted in the urine around the time of ovulation.

I don't record mucus changes on a regular basis. But,

I do use my mucus observation to substantiate what I am seeing on the temperature graph. What I am interested in doing since I have access to a microscope is to take a swab of the mucus to observe the ferning pattern. We only have 12 days in the month when we use a condom or an alternate form of love making.

ROB: As I said before, I am involved in this too. I feel that it is nice if the man is involved in the method. Some men aren't going to be into it, but that doesn't mean that the method still won't work for the woman.

JULIE: Yeah, but it sure helps if the man's into it, too.

ROB: I've told other people about it. I even told my mother. She's a medical tech and is interested in this sort of thing. I couldn't tell what her emotional reaction to the idea was, but clinically speaking she thought it was a sound idea. She didn't think that we were crazy or taking a large chance by using it. As a biochemist, it also makes sense to me in terms of what I know about female physiology.

JULIE: I feel also that the diaphragm and condom are much more inconvenient than the method. And as I have already said I don't consider using the pill as anything but dangerous, and the IUD is dangerous too. I don't find it a bother to take my temperature in the morning. It kind of gives me a chance to wake up slowly.

ROB: Yes, it's a nice interlude.

JULIE: One thing that I have found, is that my temperature will vary if I wake up two hours earlier than usual one morning. But, if that happens I just note that on my chart. If I even feel weird and my temperature seems unusual I note that on my chart. Sometimes I can't pinpoint the exact day that I ovulate, but I can always understand my chart. Some cycles, my temperature goes up a little, down, and then up in a stair-step fashion. But, I just follow the rules, and when it is up three days I am comfortable that I am safe. Then it's really nice, because I feel very free. I feel that I understand my body and what it is doing. That's perfect control of your body.

ROB: This method can even help to predict when her periods will come. She says that she never used to know when they would come, but now we can always tell. It's probably just because we are consciously following the process in an orderly way.

JULIE: Yes, what I like most is that I have a feeling about my cycle that I never had before.

You know, contraception is only needed when you are fertile and this is only one small part of the cycle. I remember that one of the first things that was brought out when I took my first course on reproduction was that other female mammals are only sexually receptive when they are fertile. But, the female human is sexually receptive almost any time. That was a big thing—a woman doesn't have sex just because some hormonal thing triggers that response. Contraception is appropriate for that time in the cycle when she is fertile, and it isn't needed for the rest of it.

I think that most anyone can use this method if they want to. You don't have to be very routinized and rigid to use the method. I'm not. Firstly, though, you have to be fed up with the chemical methods of contraception. You have to not want to change the chemistry of your body. Then you have to be interested in your cycle—to want to know about it and understand it. And then, you have to be willing to take your temperature. I think that it's no more of a pain than brushing your teeth—maybe less because you are learning something about yourself.

Pat J.

Pat is a 36-year-old Catholic, and mother of two, who has been teaching Natural Family Planning and is thoroughly sold on it. Both she and her husband believe that Natural Family Planning is right from a religious point of view and from a concern for health safety. Her thinking is both traditional and nouveau.

PAT: I am 36 and have one foot in the old Church and one foot in the new one. I must still say that in my heart, and in my husband's feelings, I have to believe in what the Pope has told me. He has spoken and said that there is no other way. I just wish that someone would tell him about this method [NBCP] so he doesn't come out and say just rhythm [Calendar Rhythm]. Rhythm has a bad name because of the failure rate, but we [our clinic] have a failure rate of about 1% using both methods [temperature and mucus]. We are basically a religious family and feel good about not doing anything artificial or against our Church. I feel better for it and I think that our marriage is stronger for it, too.

I first became interested in Natural Family Planning after the birth of our second child, in 1968. He came only 13 months after the birth of our first child, and psychologically and physically I felt that I didn't want another one. My husband agreed.

We were very pleased with having our two children and financially felt that we couldn't afford more. We had had a boy and a girl. I hate to harp on that, but the reality today is that finances are important. I wanted to give them what I could without overindulging them. I want them both to go to college if that is what they want. We're also paying off a mortgage, and my husband is the only one who works. We want to make our family happy and not have finances be another problem.

So when I went back to my obstetrician for my post-partum exam, I told him, "I can't practice Calendar Rhythm because my cycle is so erratic." I didn't want the pill for moral reasons and medical reasons, and the devices [IUDs] completely turned me off. He introduced me at that time to just the basal body temperature method. I used it for three months and he then informed me that there was a group in the area teaching this method. They had three sessions at that time, teaching the method in round table discussion, and we participated.

I took my temperature and went to these meetings. Meanwhile my husband was very skeptical. He thought that it was just Calendar Rhythm. We got completely convinced by listening to the other couples, finding out what it meant to them, and started it, and kept with it. Eventually we were so engrossed that we wanted to teach the method to other people. The obstetrician was looking for other people to help teach the method and we started doing that. We have been teaching it for four years as a couple. My husband is actually president of the board of the organization.

What I like most about the method is that it is natural. I don't have to use any devices and there are no medical problems like blood clots associated with it. I am happy with it most because it is not just my responsibility. My husband has to be involved. We have a joke between us. He has convinced me that I haven't been awake for the last seven years of taking my temperature. We wake up in the morning, he sticks the thermometer under my tongue, does his thing, and after five or ten minutes takes it out. I've never dropped it or broken it. In fact, I am still using the same thermometer. The numbers have rubbed off and rather than replacing it, I just paint it with nail polish, rub it in and just keep on using it over and over. My husband reads my graphs. I plot the temperature each morning, but he reads the charts and knows when the safe time is. I think that there is a mental thing for him, too. He doesn't have to be concerned that I am using or taking something that is potentially harmful. He loves his family, and knows that I will be healthy when he comes home.

When my children were little and started to cry, my husband got up so that I would have a basal body temperature. We discussed it and he knew that I had to have at least three hours sleep before taking my temperature. If it was real early in the morning, I would get up and have enough time to get back to sleep to take my basal temperature. If it was at four o'clock, let's say, he would get up to make sure that the baby was all right. We have three c's in our relationship, commitment, communication and consideration. And basically we are both committed to the method.

We can communicate a heck of a lot better because of it, too. I came into marriage as an only child, and had a lot to learn, and this method has helped me a lot in discussing things. I now feel that if I have to face something I can say it. That doesn't come from the liberation movement, but from just knowing that I can talk to him, and he can talk to me. Nobody flies off the handle or gets hurt by it. We both understand that we are on the method to prevent unwanted pregnancies.

That's another thing about the method. If there are any marital problems this method is not going to cure them. It actually might emphasize them a little more. There are a lot of women whose husbands refuse to do it. I can't imagine doing this without my husband going along with it. Where would I be at if I said tonight is unsafe and my husband said, "I don't care what that thing says, I don't believe it." I know of cases where the woman keeps on saying that her husband isn't into the method and she gets pregnant.

I also know of women whose husbands have thoroughly convinced them that withdrawal is safe. It is not safe. It only takes one tiny drop of sperm to make you pregnant. One drop of semen can have millions of sperm. In fact, I had a call today from a woman who thinks that she is pregnant and whose husband convinced her that withdrawal worked. That's a problem with the marriage. He's saying, "I am the man and I am the boss."

Sometimes I forget to take my temperature. My husband travels about four times a year for about three days each time. When he's not there I sometimes get up without thinking about it. I just have to make a note about it on the chart. Basically, when he is around I have never forgotten.

How we relate to the unsafe time is important, too. You can have other ways [besides intercourse] for being good to each other. You can sit down and read together, you can get into a hobby together, or spend more time with the children. For the time that you know you can't have intercourse you just throw yourself into your family life a little more. Sometimes, if I feel like doing something special around the house, like taking the house apart, I won't do it when I am safe so that I won't get real tired. My husband is so aware of my cycle that he always knows what is going on.

He also knows about the tensions just at the premenstrual time. Before I started on the method I never really knew what was causing these tensions and anxiety. I just knew that I would get very nervous, cry at the drop of a hat, or scream at the top of my lungs for no apparent reason. With the method I found out that this wasn't an abnormal thing, but something that I could learn to control if I knew it was coming and could feel that it was coming. Now he knows when it is and I know when it is and we can deal with it.

I said before that I never thought that I had regular cycles. When I first went to the doctor, I told him that my cycles were very irregular. I think that everyone thinks that if their cycle is not 28 days they're not normal. Well, normal for me is not 28 days, but 31 to 35 days. With this Calendar Rhythm didn't work. It was always too long or too short. Now I've noticed that around age 30 I came down to a cycle of 28 or 29 days. Once in a while I may have a short cycle, 24 days, but then the next cycle is a little longer, around 31 or 32 days. It averages out. I now know that everyone has their own pattern. I can recognize my graphs out of a pile of graphs very easily.

We started using the mucus [Billings] method in our clinic about two years ago. What it is, is just keeping track of the mucus secretions in the vagina, at different times during the cycle. Some women chime in right away that they discharge every day. That's not what we're looking for.

Prior to ovulation you have a dry feeling or sensation on the lips of the vagina. Then you change to a cloudy thick mucus plug that is yellowish in color. Then, it changes to a real clear, smooth, watery stretchy one like that of the uncooked white of an egg. This is the peak symptom and corresponds to the time just before ovulation. It then tapers off and disappears entirely, or it may get sticky and cloudy again. What is important is that you get to recognize the peak symptom.

What made me realize that this wasn't Calendar Rhythm and what appealed to me at first was the number of safe days. If you are using the Calendar Rhythm method you lose a whole other week. Using the Billings method you can be sure about the preovulatory safe time. You know, I don't ever mind the routine, and in fact now I am lost if I don't take my temperature in the morning. When we go on vacation my thermometer goes with me. This last summer I went away without my thermometer on purpose. I had just started my period and knew exactly where I was at in terms of my cycle. I used the Billings method and things went just great. It all kind of clicked together and I knew that you could use one method alone. I still prefer to do both and use one as a check on the other.

I think that everyone can use the method. Women who are going through the change [menopause] cannot use the temperature method since their temperatures are very erratic. But, they can use the Billings method. Nursing mothers can use the Billings method too, since they will not have a temperature pattern defined by ovulation [they're not necessarily ovulating yet], but they can use the secretion method. A woman with an irregular cycle is actually better off with this method, since she will know when she is ovulating and be more relaxed about her cycle.

My daughter knows where I am at with this thing, too. There's no getting away from it. She's 9½ and beginning to ask questions, and I'll tell you one thing that is great is that for all women who have gone through this, they know a lot more about their body because of it. Now I can start telling my daughter about it, and feel that I have no hangups in talking about it. She knows that she can ask anything that she wants, and I try and answer her in terms that she will understand.

I have begun to prepare her, because she is starting to show some maturing, and I plan on starting her on the method as soon as she starts having menstrual cycles. I think that teenage girls should be taking their temperatures and that we should teach it in schools in sex education classes. I prefer seeing a 15-year-old taking her temperature than taking the pill. There's a chance that she might sterilize herself by taking the pill and be miserable when she's 26 and wants to have a family. Nobody really knows what the pill is going to do. The reality is that women are fertile only certain times and coping with that is an education.

Anna O.

Anna O. is 32 years old and a Physician's Assistant student. Her husband is a builder and they have one child. They are both interested in this birth control method. Anna uses the method even though she had an unwanted pregnancy with it. She began using it as her sole method of birth control before becoming really certain of how it works. Now she feels that this was due to a combination of inadequate teaching (or lack of understanding) and the fact that she didn't observe her cycles for six months before actually using the method. She still feels that it is a safe and reliable form of birth control and as a person interested in medicine she feels that she will use it in birth control counseling. She does think, however, that it is important that people who use Natural Family Planning be "careful people," and emphasizes the need for caution in beginning to use the program as one's sole method of contraception.

ANNA: I am 32 years old and have been married for five years. My occupation now is that of a student, soon to become a Physician's Assistant. I have one child who is four years old and have been with my husband for six years. We plan on having another child in a couple of years.

The reason that I became interested in Natural Family Planning was due to total exasperation with other methods of birth control. I had taken birth control pills on and off for several years, interspersing their use with an IUD. I had unpleasant side effects from birth control pills, such as chronic yeast infections and weight gain. I always felt uneasy about putting these foreign chemicals in my body and would only take them for a year or a year and a half and then stop. The main problem with the IUD was that I had more pain and much more bleeding with my period. The last time I had an IUD it got embedded in my uterus and the extraction was very painful. I had a lot of bleeding and it took me a week to recover from it.

After that I decided to try a diaphragm, which I had never used before. The problem with the diaphragm was that I have a retroverted uterus and it was very difficult to insert and almost impossible to take out. It was so difficult to remove that once I left it in for a couple of days and could not get it out by myself. I finally had to have my husband remove it, which was very painful. And a few days later, I got a very bad urinary tract infection, which I am convinced was due to the traumatic removal of the diaphragm. This took two months to clear up because I was allergic to several of the medications, and one of the medicines didn't work at all. After all of this I was really exasperated.

We started using prophylactics—rubbers—for several months until a friend conveyed the information about Natural Family Planning. She asked me if I would want to take a course in it and learn about it. I was very interested. The idea of not putting any chemicals or anything foreign into my body was very exciting to me. So I started using the basal body temperature method a little over a year ago. I also tried to use the mucus method a month later when it was taught in the course. It was during the second month using this method that I became pregnant. I had just started taking my temperature the month before and averaging the mean estrogenic and progesterone temperatures hadn't been explained well enough to me. So when my temperature went up and down during the month I thought that I was having an anovulatory cycle. I had been taught that a woman has an anovulatory cycle once every 12 or 18 months, and when the second month didn't show a clear cut temperature rise like the month before, I thought "ah, ha, I didn't ovulate this month." We didn't take any precautions after the 18th day of my cycle and as a result I became pregnant.

When I went back to the class I said to the doctor, "Look at my graph, I didn't ovulate this month." He said, "oh, yes you did, you ovulated right here." I couldn't see it from my graph since there were so many spikes in it. The temperature had gone up and down, varying about 5 tenths of a degree from day to day. I hadn't thought that there could be such a wide variation in temperatures during a normal cycle. I feel that this was a problem of poor presentation or lack of understanding on my part, and that no one should use this method exclusively for the first six months, or until they thoroughly understand it. You should use some method of contraception or take some kind of precaution until you feel comfortable with the system. After that you will have enough observations to look back and be able to see when you ovulate from month to month. I did not have a desire to get pregnant at the time. It was a lack of understanding about the method.

After I had the abortion I was very scared about becoming pregnant again. I thought about going back to birth control pills, but I really didn't want that. I decided to try Natural Family Planning again, being extremely careful. At first I mainly was taking my temperature, while using prophylactics most of the time.

Using the BBT method has put me more in touch with my body. I began to notice a slight lower abdominal pain around the time of ovulation that goes on for one to three days. I have probably always had such a pain around the time of ovulation, but never correlated the two before. Now I can use it as another indication that ovulation has or is about to occur.

I was very careful using the temperature method for about three months after my abortion. After seeing the variations in my cycle for a while I became more confident about the method again. Now, because I know that my cycle varies from 28 to 32 days I don't use birth control for the first nine days. During the unsafe time we use abstinence or a precaution until my temperature has remained elevated for three days.

It's all pretty easy now. My husband and I alternate getting up in the morning with our child. But, if it's my turn and my son wakes up while I am taking my temperature, my husband will take care of him until I am finished. Although the abortion was a very painful and traumatic experience, I still feel that Natural Family Planning is an adequate and safe method of birth control. However, after the experience of an abortion, I still get worried if my period is a little later than usual.

This happens even if my temperature chart definitely shows that I have ovulated for that month.

I don't think that I will ever use an IUD again. But, if I did get pregnant using Natural Family Planning again it might make me want to use the birth control pill. I know that if that happened I would be so upset that I would want something that I thought would be 100% safe. I do think that people can use Natural Family Planning if they are conscientious people, and understand the method well before actually using it as a method of birth control.

CHAPTER ELEVEN

A Doctor's View of the New Birth Control Program

James P. Furlong is a doctor who specializes in obstetrics and gynecology. He has been a proponent and teacher of Sympto-thermic birth control for many years, and has helped us greatly in our efforts to write this book. In addition to his active private practice, he teaches Natural Family Planning at the Family Life Information Center in Albany, New York.

What follows is a conversation we had recently with Dr. Furlong about the New Birth Control Program.

CHRIS: When did you start teaching Natural Family Planning?

DR. FURLONG: I started teaching Sympto-thermic rhythm [the forerunner of Natural Family Planning] approximately 20 years ago. The course has been enlarged and extended to include the mucus [Billings] method and Keefe's cervical method. All told we've taught 830 couples up to the present. Some of the women are single, and some come without their husbands because the men are working, or just refuse to come. We've even had one communal group comprised of five women and three men, who wanted to practice Natural Family Planning.

CHRIS: What seems to make the program work best?

DR. FURLONG: The whole program seems to work better in a compatible family setting. What I am saying is that it works better if the husband understands it. We often get converts. Some men come reluctantly at first and then change their minds.

I advise women to learn all they can about themselves, and I don't like to call this a method of contraception. I like to call it a method of fertility control. It's different. Contraception means using something to alter. This method means letting your body know when you are fertile and when you are not.

CHRIS: What do you think about the oral contraceptive pill?

DR. FURLONG: I have personal objections to the pill. I am basically a naturalist, and I have always felt that anything you do to alter mother nature has a tendency to cost. The cost can be a little or the cost can be a lot. In some people the cost has been very great. Almost every day that you pick up the paper there is something new that is directly caused by the pill. Big things that we see are pulmonary emboli [blood clots in the lungs], sudden onset of complete and irreversible blindness, strokes; and a brand new thing in the last year, for women who have taken the pill for six or seven years, is large, encapsulated, bleeding liver tumors.

The cost here would seem to be too great. However, these severe or serious complications of taking the pill do not occur very often. They only occur in about one in 500,000 people. So not many women have these severe diseases, but the ones who do are in great trouble.

I do not agree with the argument that it is safer to take the pill than to get pregnant. Maternal morbidity and mortality figures are misleading. Any accident that happens to a woman from the time she gets pregnant until she is six weeks past having her child is put down as maternal morbidity or mortality. If a woman were to fall out of a second story window and kill herself landing on a sidewalk when her baby is five weeks old, that's maternal mortality. I have great difficulty equating the pill with pregnancy. Pregnancy is positive, the pill is negative. If one could control their fertility without using the pill then there would be no morbidity or mortality due to the pill.

CHRIS: How successful is your group in using Natural Family Planning?

DR. FURLONG: As far as we know now we are running about a 1% failure rate in methodology [of Natural Family Planning]. That is the method fails about 1% of the time. People have a tendency to fail a lot more than methods. We have people get pregnant who know full well that they should not have had intercourse at the time, but they do. It isn't generally due to lack of communication between the couple, but due to an indecisive feeling about their family size. Natural Family Planning works best with people who have a purpose for not having children at the moment. A person who gets pregnant is generally one who is conflicted about pregnancy to begin with.

We don't have statistics on user failure. But most of the cause for user failure is a person who knows they shouldn't but goes ahead and does anyway. We have had several failures when they've used mechanical contraception that failed. It was during a time when they shouldn't have had intercourse, so I don't think that this method should be blamed for that failure.

CHRIS: What factors do you find help make a couple successful with Natural Family Planning?

DR. FURLONG: Age seems to be a factor. A person approaching forty who has decided "that's my family" seems to be the most motivated, and the method works very well there. Economic status doesn't seem to play a role. The longer the couple is married seems to coincide with being satisfied about family size, and for these couples the method works very well.

Most people who come to us have already made up their minds and decided that they want to use the method. I think that finding us has been a problem. We need more publicity. I think that there are more people who would like to try Natural Family Planning. These are people who have been afraid of the pill and IUDs, or have been on them and are afraid and want to get off.

CHRIS: How does the pill affect your temperature?

DR. FURLONG: It varies so much how long you have to wait coming off the pill before you see a good temperature cycle. It is very much like coming off of pregnancy. It may take two or three months to get straightened out, or it may go immediately like just before, with a 28 day cycle. But, the most common thing coming off the pill is to be a week, ten days or two weeks late.

The temperature will always reflect the physiology. A woman will have a flat temperature graph until she ovulates. It may be ten days late or whatever her pattern is. We have women practicing taking their temperatures while they are on the pill. They will have their rise around Day 5 when they begin taking the progesterol [in the pill], and then it remains up.

CHRIS: Would you please explain how the mucus method works for an average woman?

DR. FURLONG: Taking our hypothetical 28 or 29 Day cycle, Day 1 is the beginning of the menstrual cycle and the onset of bleeding. From Day 5 to about Day 8 the vagina is relatively dryer. On about Day 9 the cervix puts out a real thick, sticky, stringy, shiny, usually cloudy, mucus plug. Rapidly, within 12 hours or so, it becomes thin, watery, very slippery and very stretchy.

On Day 14, approximately, the woman ovulates. The mucus drainage decreases over the next two days, and on about Day 17 the vagina becomes relatively dryer again. The vagina is never really dry, but it is not slippery. During the dry days from Day 5 to Day 8, and from Day 17 to Day 28, the pH in the vagina is approximately 4.5 [acid]. The pH of 4.5 is detrimental to the life of sperm and their motility [ability to swim]. It kills them usually within two hours. Once the mucus plug has come out of the cervix, the vagina is changed to a pH of around 7. This is conducive to the life and transport of sperm. It makes them live longer, swim farther and swim faster. And they will survive for as many days as they are exposed to this friendly medium.

CHRIS: Is the menstrual period safe for unprotected intercourse?

DR. FURLONG: Having sexual relations during the menses is not safe according to the Billings method. This can produce unexpected pregnancies. If a woman were unfortunate enough to have a twenty-one day cycle and an 8-day period, she would ovulate the day before her period stopped. And if she were to have intercourse any time that the mucus was present, say four to five days prior to the 7th, pregnancy could very well occur. The reason why it is not safe with the mucus method is that the mucus drainage would be covered up by the menstrual bleeding, and there would be no way to tell that it was there.

The other way that pregnancy can occur during the bleeding is that every once in a while you see a woman who is having her period every two weeks. She has bleeding for five days, and then two weeks later she has bleeding for four days. What she is doing is having her period and then having ovulatory bleeding, later in the cycle. Occasionally the estrogen level will drop so much during ovulation that bleeding occurs. The lining of the uterus thinks that the woman is beginning her cycle and she starts to bleed. Within a day or so the estrogen level rises up quickly again and the bleeding stops, and sort of a brownish drainage goes on for two or three days.

Now if you use this time for having intercourse you would say that this is the first day of my period, and really it would be the first day of ovulation. The menstrual discharge is alkaline (pH approximately 7) and is conducive to the life of sperm. If you were to ovulate very soon after the end of your menses there might not be any dry days. In fact, there wouldn't be any according to Billings.

CHRIS: What kind of response have you had with the mucus method?

DR. FURLONG: The mucus method has veen very successful. Young women seem to understand it and be able to interpret the system better than women over forty. I think that this may be because they are more open people. The vagina is not a bad place, and mucus is not a bad thing. Older people, when they were young, will tell you that you just didn't talk about these things. We have been teaching this method to lactating [breast-feeding] women as well. The lactating women and the premenopausal women are exactly the same in the mucus method. According to the information that we have so far, fertility is always accompanied by a vaginal discharge [mucus] that is thin, watery, clear and especially slippery and stretchy. This mucus, when put between two fingers, will stretch out four or five inches. The nonfertile mucus will stretch only half an inch. I think that women do best if they know both systems—temperature and mucus—and this goes for premenopausal and lactating women, too.

CHRIS: Please describe the cervical changes that you teach women to look for.

DR. FURLONG: Keefe is a doctor in New York, who in about 1960, took 20 nurses who knew what they were doing and studied the changes in their cervix throughout the menstrual cycle. He built for them a special speculum. It was a stainless steel pipe about six inches long with a mirror and a light on the end of it. Every day these women would go into the bathroom, put one foot up on the edge of a tub, put the speculum into their vagina, and observe what was going on with their cervix.

After several years of working with this they found that there was a well-defined pattern. When the woman was *not* fertile the cervix was lower, firm, about the same consistency as the end of the nose, closed and dry. When the woman was fertile, the cervix was higher, considerably so, softer and much more like the upper lip than the end of the nose. It was also open, and the big thing is that it was wet and slippery.

The mucus that appears wet and slippery at the opening of the vagina comes from the cervix. So, by putting two fingers into the vagina and feeling the end of the cervix you know hours ahead that you have or have not started to have this fertile mucus. The cervix should be checked the same time each day under the same circumstances. For instance, you shouldn't check it right after having a bowel movement one day and not the other days.

KEEFE'S CERVICAL CHANGES

Fertile/Not Safe for Intercourse cervix is high			Not fertile/Safe for Intercourse cervix is lower		
ʋ	ʋ	soft (like your lip)	ʋ	ʋ	firm (like your nose)
ʋ	ʋ	open (to a fingertip)	ʋ	ʋ	closed
ʋ	ʋ	wet	ʋ	ʋ	dryer
ʋ	ʋ	slippery (mucus)	ʋ	ʋ	not slippery (mucus)

CHRIS: How do you teach the method in your clinic?

DR. FURLONG: We teach the method in four sessions. This includes a complete physical, pelvic exam and lab work at the end. The first session is a lecture on anatomy and physiology, and an introduction to the thermic changes in the body (the temperature method). This includes an explanation of the graph, and a film on the physiology of human reproduction.

The second session is a film with Dr. Billings. We also explain the Billings method, and go over the temperature method again. We also read each chart, so each person knows what their chart means. The third session is a round-table discussion of things that we have done up to that point. And the fourth session is the physical exam.

Sympto-thermia was a term coined in the late 1950's for temperature and any of the signs that women get before ovulation—like pain in the side, frequency or urgency or urination, or changes in mood. Billings' mucus method is newer. The whole thing is called Natural Family Planning.

Methods of detecting ovulation are coming off the press so fast that we can't even keep up with them. Lots and lots of people have suddenly become interested in normal physiology. I think that before long we will have other reliable tests. Right now we teach the physiology of the female body, and how to detect its change with temperature, mucus, and Keefe's cervical change methods.

CHAPTER TWELVE

A Psychologist's Perspective of the New Birth Control Program

Dr. Joseph E. Bernier is an Assistant Professor in the Department of Counselling Psychology at the State University of New York, in Albany. He received his Ph.D. from the University of Minnesota and now has a special interest in problems of human development and marriage and family therapy. He is the author of several articles and books in counselor education and human development.

We asked Dr. Bernier for his opinion of the New Birth Control Program and of this book. Here's what he said:

I have been asked by the authors to respond to the contraception program they outline in this manual. After reading the manuscript, I find myself generally enthusiastic about the potential "psychological pay-offs" inherent in this "new" method. At the same time I am not without some words of caution. I would like to take this opportunity to share some of these reactions with you.

Cultivating Individual Differences and Self-Management
Generally speaking, the New Birth Control Program (NBCP) has important implications for the development of self-awareness and self-control; that is, for our

desire to learn more about ourselves, have choices, and manage our lives. First, NBCP has the potential to assist each woman in the growing awareness of her sexuality. The term "sexuality" is used in its broadest sense and encompasses sexual physiology, associated moods and emotions, energy level, etc., in short, many of those physical or "mental" factors that are associated with a woman's sexual functioning.

While birth control pills have without a doubt successfully managed to regulate or control women's menstrual cycles, one broad side-effect has been to reduce or wipe out some of the differences between women in terms of their menstrual cycle. In addition, the regulation of a woman's cycle through medication has reduced the natural month-to-month (but often predictable) fluctuations found in many women. In sum, while effectively preventing pregnancy, the pill has had the effect of minimizing individual differences between women and within any one woman.

On the other hand, although not chemically reducing these individual differences, other common contraceptive practices, such as the condom, diaphragm, spermicidal creams, calendar rhythm, complete abstinence from intercourse, and even abortion have done little to increase a woman's awareness of her bodily functioning. In other words, they have not encouraged women to monitor their sexual physiology and behavior.

The New Birth Control Program offers an alternative to these pitfalls by providing women with a basis for understanding the physiology of reproduction and predicting their own menstrual rhythms. The avenue for this self-knowledge and prediction is through observing and graphing your daily body temperature and the changes in vaginal position and secretion. As you have seen, these are the primary techniques of NBCP.

Psychology's interest (especially the applied clinical specialties) in self-observation and charting (graphing) procedures is on the rise, and thus NBCP appears consistent with innovative approaches to developing self-knowledge, personal management, and self-change.[1] The "psychological use" of charting one's thoughts, feelings, and behavior has proven very versatile and the application of these procedures to the area of sexual functioning seems no less powerful. For example, as is discussed by the authors, beyond plotting your physiological and anatomical changes you may want to also monitor (observe and graph) the emotions you experience each day of your cycle, your energy level, desire for sex, general outlook on life, and the fluctuations in your attitudes toward significant other people. The list of things to observe and graph is almost endless and after a while you may notice some interesting patterns developing in association with or maybe even apart from your sexual anatomical/physiological change.[2]

An additional "plus" for NBCP is that it may have some potential for freeing women to "love" their bodies. It seems to me that some women approach contraception in a "me against my body" fashion—that is, their capacity to conceive is viewed as a "curse" which warrants absolute suppression and control by taking in "foreign" substances such as the pill, an IUD, a diaphragm and jellies. While respecting one's power to conceive, NBCP encourages women to "listen to" or "get in touch with" their bodies by carefully monitoring bodily changes. This may enable or encourage women to adopt a loving and respectful "me with my body" attitude.

---

[1]For further information on self-management techniques in psychology please consult:

1) Watson, D.L. and Tharp, R.G. *Self-Directed Behavior: Self Modification for Personal Adjustment*, Monterey, Calif.: Brooks/Cole Publishing Co., 1972.

2) Lazarus, A.A. and Fay, A. *I Can If I Want To.* N.Y.: Wm. Morrow, Inc. 1975.

3) Foster, C. *Developing Self-Control.* Kalamazoo, Michigan: Behaviordelia, Inc., 1974.

[2]Men may also get into the swing of things and chart their own "cycles" —that is, their energy level, feelings, moods, etc.—and compare these with their sexual mates.

In sum, by adopting the New Birth Control Program women may obtain a better understanding of female sexuality in general and come to a greater awareness and respect of themselves as sexual beings. Unlike other birth control methods, NBCP allows for individual differences, while enhancing a woman's understanding of her unique or idiosyncratic sexual functioning. Depending on how many psychological factors she chooses to monitor in addition to the required body temperature and shifts in cervical position and mucus, she may begin to gain an increased awareness and understanding of the complex interrelationships between sexual-physical and sexual-mental functioning.

In addition, the information obtained through self-observation and graphing may help a woman in educating her partner about her sexual physiology and associated moods, attitudes, and energy level.

All this however underscores the need for mutual caring and effective communication between partners—a topic to be taken up later.

Precautionary Words

Through this book, Hank Pizer and Christine Garfink provide you with the technical "know-how" to begin the New Birth Control Program. In addition, the technological hardware—that is, the basal thermometer and special graphs—are presently available and can be easily obtained. However, neither the authors nor the pharmacist can provide you with the motivation to use this knowledge and equipment properly. Here lies the major thrust of those concerns and cautions I mentioned earlier.

Although the issue of motivation is very complex, research data obtained through a survey of couples using NBCP suggest two general areas for comment and consideration. First concerns a woman's attitudes toward her sexuality and her role in relation to men. As previously discussed, the New Birth Control Program involves careful self-observation and the precise use of graphs. While these skills are not difficult to learn and use, they do require some diligence, careful attention, and commitment to the program. Without these basic ingredients, you may be setting yourself up for failure in preventing pregnancy.

In addition to the use of observation and graphs, NBCP women must refrain from unprotected intercourse during their "unsafe" or fertile days. Survey results tell us that some women and many men find this "requirement" difficult and problematic. Some individuals appear reluctant to abstain from unprotected intercourse because of their distaste for other contraceptive methods and/or the narrow range of sexual behavior they consider appropriate and satisfying. However, in light of this information, it is particularly important for women using NBCP to view themselves as "in charge of" or directly responsible for their own sexuality. This calls for a kind of self-confidence and assertiveness many women find difficult to muster up.[3]

While we could speculate on the many reasons for a woman's lack of assertiveness and confidence, we must keep two points in mind. First, women have inherited a legacy of time-honored passivity and self-sacrifice which has been acted out in their sexual relationships. Secondly, some of the most basic "rules" ("shoulds") that govern our relationships are often passed on from generation to generation and are first learned by watching how our mothers reacted to our fathers and vice versa.

What all this means is that women (and men) have a social, cultural, and psychological heritage that exerts some influence on how they relate sexually.[4] However, women (and men) need not be captives of their psychological and social histories. They do, in fact, have some choice in this matter. The point is that the po-

---

[3]Please note that many men also lack assertive behavior and feelings of confidence.
[4]This is not intended to minimize the significant role played by situational factors operating in the present.

tential NBCP user must honestly consider how she relates to men, take an inventory of her "sexual shoulds," and determine whether she has the desire, know-how, and strength to "take charge" of her sexual behavior and the proper use of NBCP. For some women, the responsible use of NBCP may require that they "shake" old habits and learn new ways of relating to men and their own sexuality.

The second area for comment focuses on the quality of the relationships that exist between NBCP women and their male partners. The survey data mentioned earlier seems to suggest that the *optimal* NBCP relationship is built upon a foundation of trust, cooperation, similarity of sexual values, and open and clear communication—all of which have stood the test of time for the couple.

The value or desirability of these qualities may seem to be obvious or common sense and certainly not restricted to NBCP couples. However, logic tells us that they are more crucial for NBCP users than for women who take the pill or use an IUD, precisely because of the daily "demands" inherent in NBCP use. In addition, these comments are not intended to discourage the woman who does not have a regular sexual partner from using NBCP. In fact, as is pointed out in the text, the New Birth Control Program offers several advantages to the woman who has infrequent sexual involvements. Nonetheless, some of these women may find their jobs a bit tougher in the face of potential demanding, uncooperative, and uncommitted sexual partners. For example, if an NBCP woman has just recently become involved with a man who she enjoys, she might find it difficult to limit or adjust her sexual activities during ovulation. In this instance, depending on her partner's attitudes, she may view the future of their relationship to be dependent, in part, on their having regular intercourse. If, for whatever reason, she feels unable to discuss their relationship and sexual practices with her partner, she may find herself caught in a bind with high stakes for everyone concerned. This example serves to illustrate the advantages of having a solid relationship serve as the foundation for the New Birth Control Program. Of course, the building of such a relationship is no easy task and may require that sexual partners learn new ways to talk and relate to each other.[5]

In conclusion, by writing this epilogue I am not attesting to the effectiveness of NBCP in preventing pregnancy. Research data is available that specifically addresses this issue. The authors of this manual do summarize some of this information for you. However, I have attempted to anticipate and sketch some of the psychological ramifications (the psychological prerequisites and potential side effects) of the New Birth Control Program. I hope that my discussion will prove useful to you in reading this manual and in choosing a method of birth control that suits your unique needs and preferences. Although probably not suited for everywoman, the method taught through this manual may be appropriate for you.

Read the manual, explore the alternatives, and form a decision based on your life circumstances and tastes.

Joseph E. Bernier, Ph.D.
Assistant Professor
Department of Counseling
    and Personnel Psychology
State University of New York at Albany

---

[5]For those couples who are interested in improving their relationship, I recommend that you read:

1) Satir, V. *Peoplemaking*. Palo Alto, Calif.: Science and Behavior Books, 1972.

2) Satir, V. *Making Contact*. Millbrae, Calif.: Celestial Arts Publishers, 1975. (An abbreviated version of *Peoplemaking*)

3) Ellis, T. and Harper, R. *A Guide to Successful Marriage*. No. Hollywood, Calif.: Willshire Press, 1975.

APPENDICES

Glossary

Abstinence: Refraining from sexual intercourse; or a period of time when one does not engage in sexual intercourse.

Acid: Chemically opposite to alkaline substances. Acid substances are generally sour to the taste, such as vinegar (acetic acid), lemon juice (citric acid), etc. An acid vagina is not a favorable environment for sperm.

Alkaline: Basic, or chemically opposite to acid substances. Some alkaline substances are lye (sodium hydroxide) and bicarbonate of soda. As the vagina changes from acid towards mildly basic, it becomes a more favorable environment for sperm.

Amenorrhea: Failure to menstruate; i.e., not having a period.

Anovulatory cycle: A menstrual month in which there is no ovulation. During this time a woman is not fertile.

Anteverted uterus: A uterus that is tipped forward in the pelvis. This is considered a normal variation of the female anatomy unless unfavorable symptoms occur.

Artifact: An artificial or somehow unreliable reading.

Basal body temperature: The temperature of your body at rest. The temperature represents your baseline metabolism.

Biphasic curve: A graph with two phases. In this con-

text a biphasic curve has a lower preovulatory level
and a higher postovulatory level.

Calendar rhythm: The use of the days of the month to
predict when it is safe or unsafe to have unprotected
sexual relations.

Cervix: The neck of an organ. The neck of the uterus is
the *cervix uteri*.

Clitoris: A small organ located under the anterior part
of the labia minora in the female; it is anatomically
homologous to the penis of the male. The clitoris is
sexually sensitive and engorges with blood during
stimulation.

Condom: A synthetic or natural sheath placed over the
penis before sexual intercourse to prevent sperm
from gaining entrance to the vagina. It is a male form
of contraception.

Diaphragm: A flexible, cuplike piece of plastic or rub-
ber that fits over the cervix. When used with a sperm-
acide it is a female form of contraception.

Egg: The woman's sex or germ cell, which is produced
by the ovary during ovulation.

Ejaculation: The expulsion of semen (including sperm)
from the male during sexual excitement.

Endometrium: The vascular lining of the uterus of the
female. The superficial layer is shed during a normal menstrual cycle.

Estrogen: A female sex hormone, produced by the
ovaries, that is responsible for the development of
female sex characteristics.

Fallopian tube: The tube that connect the ovary to the
uterus. It is a conduit through which the egg passes
from the ovary, where it is produced, to the uterus.

Ferning: A pattern of mucus when seen under mag-
nification. Fertile mucus has a characteristic pattern
like that of ferns in the woods.

Fertility: The ability to produce offspring.

Fertilization: The uniting of sperm and egg to produce
a human embryo.

Hormone: A chemical produced by an organ of the

body and carried by the bloodstream to another part of the body, where it stimulates a certain response. Hormones control many of our most important body functions; they include such substances as estrogen, progesterone, cortisol, thyroxine, growth hormone, and so on.

Infection: The invasion of the body by a harmful organism, which under certain conditions multiplies in the body and produces harmful effects.

IUD: Intrauterine device; a metallic or plastic device that is inserted into the uterus as a female form of contraception.

Labia: The lips of the vulva. There are two distinct sets of labia: the labia majora are the outer structures surrounding the vaginal opening, and the labia minora are the inner structures.

Menopause: The time when menstruation ceases. More commonly considered a period of time when the menstrual periods become lighter and occur farther apart.

Menses: Menstruation:

Menstruation: This discharge through the vagina of a bloody fluid that is actually the superficial lining of the uterus. It occurs with regularity in women from puberty until fertility is terminated.

Metabolism: The total of all the energy building up and breaking down within the body. The digestion of food into usable energy units, the burning of those units during exercise, the energy required to maintain life, and the production of structural substances in the body that we see as growth are all actions of our metabolism.

Mittelschmerz: A pain felt by some women in the lower abdomen around midcycle that occurs during ovulation.

Monophasic curve: A temperature curve that does not have lower preovulatory and higher postovulatory levels. It is generally a see-saw graph.

Mucus: The secretion from the glands of the cervix;

cervical mucus changes during the menstrual cycle.

Os: The opening of the cervix, which allows menstrual blood and secretions to pass from the uterus into the vagina, and allows sperm to pass from the vagina into the uterus.

Ovaries: The female sex organs, homologous to the male testes, that produce eggs and also the female sex hormones progesterone and estrogen.

Ovulation: The development and expulsion of an egg from the female ovary. Ovulation is a complex and cyclic phenomenon controlled by hormones. It occurs approximately 14 days before the beginning of the next menstrual period.

Ovum: The female egg, or reproductive cell. When penetrated by a single sperm, it can produce an embryo.

Progesterone: A female sex hormone produced in the ovary and responsible for readying the uterus to receive and implant the fertilized egg, the development of the placenta, and the development of the mammary glands in the breast.

Retroverted uterus: A uterus that is tipped backward in the pelvis. This is considered a normal variation of the female anatomy unless unfavorable symptoms occur.

Safe day: A day when unprotected sexual intercourse will not result in fertilization, determined by basal body temperature or mucus symptoms.

Sperm: The man's sex or germ cell, produced by the testes and capable of producing an embryo when it penetrates and fertilizes the egg.

Spinnbarkheit: The stretchability of cervical mucus.

Urethra: The canal that connects the bladder to the external world and allows urine to flow out of the body.

Uterus: The womb; the female organ that holds and supplies nourishment to the developing fetus.

Viscosity: The stickiness and tackiness of a fluid.

References

Austin, C.R. Sperm fertility, viability and persistance in the female tract. *J. of Repr. Fertil.*, Suppl. 22, 1975, 75-89.

Bartzen, Peter. Effectiveness of the temperature rhythm system of contraception. *Fertil and Steril*, 18, 694, 1967.

Bilings, E., Billings, J., et. al. Symptoms and hormonal changes accompanying ovulation. *Lancet*, Feb. 1972, 282-84.

Billings, J. *Natural Family Planning*. Liturgical Press, 1975, Collegeville, Minn.

Boston Women's Health Book Collective. *Our Bodies Ourselves*. Simon and Schuster, 1976, New York.

Brayer, F. Calendar rhythm and menstrual cycle range. *Fertil, Steril*, 20, 2, 1969, 279-88.

Cohen, M. et. al. Spinnbarkeit: a characteristic of cervical mucus; significance at ovulation time. *Fertil, Steril* 3: 201-09, May-June, 1952.

Duffy, B. and Wallace, M. *Biological and medical aspects of contraception*. Univ. of Notre Dame Press, 1969, Notre Dame.

Elstein, M. and Moghissi, K., et. al. *Cervical mucus in human reproduction*. World Health Organization, Scriptor, Copenhagen, 1973.

France, J. et. al. The detection of ovulation in humans and its application in contraception. *J. Repr. Fertil*, Suppl. 22, 1975, 107-20.

Gough, H. A factor analysis of contraceptive preferences. *J. of Psychol.* 92, Jan. 76, 109-12.

Iffy, L. and Wingate. Risks of rhythm method of birth control. *The J. of Repr. Med.*, 5, 3, 1970, 11-15.

Johansson, E. et. al. Monophasic basal body temperature in ovulatory menstrual cycles. *Am. J. Obstet Gynecol.* 113, Aug. 72, 933-37.

Kar, S. Individual aspirations as related to early and late acceptance of contraception. *J. of Soc. Psych.* 83, 1971, 235-45.

Keefe, E. Self-observation of the cervix to distinguish days of possible fertility. *Bull of the Sloane Hosp. for Women,* 8, Winter, 1962, 129-136.

Keefer, Chester. *Human Ovulation.* Little, Brown and Co., 1965, Boston.

Kutner, J. A survey of fear of pregnancy and depression. *J. of Psych,* 79, 1971, 263-272.

Lacey, Louise. *Lunaception.* Warner Books, 1976, New York.

Letter: Natural Family Planning. *Lancet,* 2, Sept. 76, 579.

Lidz, R. Emotional factors in the success of contraception. *Fertil Steril.* 20, 1969, 761-71.

Lundy, J. Some personality correlates of contraceptive use among unmarried female college students. *J. Psychol.,* 80, 1972, 9-14.

Marshall, J. A field trial of the basal body temperature method of regulating births. *Lancet,* 11, 1968, 8.

Marshall, J. and Rowe, B. The effect of personal factors on the use of the basal body temperature method of regulating births. *Fertil, Steril,* 23, 6, 1972, 417-21.

Marshall, J. and Rowe, B. Psychological aspects of the basal body temperature method of regulating births. *Fertil, Steril,* 21, 1, 1970, 14-19.

Moghissi, K. Accuracy of basal body temperature for ovulation. *Fertil, Steril,* 27, 2, 1976, 207.

Moore, W. Evaluation of fertility control by periodic abstinence. *Practitioner,* 205, 1970, 38-43.

Morris, N. et al. Temporal relationship between basal body temperature nadir and LH surge in normal women. *Fertil, Steril,* 27, 7, 1976, 780-83.

Nofziger, M. *A cooperative method of natural birth control.* The Book Publishing Co., 1976, Summertown, Tenn.

Porter, J. The rhythm method of contraception. *J. Rep. Fertil,* Supp 22, 1975, 91-105.

Rosenblum, Art et. al. *The Natural Birth Control Book.* Aquarian Research Foundation, 1976, Philadelphia.

Schneider, S. et al. Repeat aborters. *Am. J. of Ob/ Gyn.* 126, 1976, 316.

Tietze, C. Mortality associated with the control of fertility. *Fam. Plann. Perspect.,* 8, 1, Jan. 76, 6-14.

Tietze, C. and Potter, R. Statistical evaluation of the rhythm method. *Am J. of Ob/Gyn.* 84, 1962, 692.

Timby, B. Ovulation method of birth control. *Am. J. of Nurs.* 76, 6, Jun. 76, 928.

Uricchio, W. and Williams, M. *Proceedings of a research conference on natural family planning.* The Human Life Foundation, 1973, Washington, D.C.

Weissman, M., et al. A trial of the ovulation method of family planning in Tonga. *Lancet,* 11, Oct., 1972, 813-816.

Wood. Emotional attitudes to contraceptive methods. *Contraception,* 2, 2, 1970, 113-126.

Zuspan, K. and Zuspan, F. Thermogenic alterations in the woman. Basal body, afternoon and bedtime temperatures. *Am. J. of Ob/Gyn.* 120, 4, 1974, 441-45.

Zuspan, F. and Rao, P. Thermogenic alterations in the woman I. Interaction of amines, ovulation and basal body temperature. *Am. J. Ob/Gyn.* 118, Mar 74, 671-8.

On Using This Book

This book was designed as a teaching manual. We have tried to make it as straightforward, clear and complete as possible. Yet in any new endeavor questions and problems inevitably arise that need explanation from a person with prior experience. Thus, *THE NEW BIRTH CONTROL PROGRAM* is a book that works best when used in conjunction with an already existing course in Natural Family Planning.

We began on our own, but learned a great deal from the Family Life Information Center in Albany, New York. There Dr. Furlong and members of his group presented the course over a four-month period and were available for questions on a regular basis. They realized correctly that in any learning process it takes time to absorb and appreciate the new material. We now feel that learning this new birth control program over a prolonged stretch, with trained people available for answering questions, is clearly the best approach. No book can fully replace a good teacher.

Below we have listed some centers where you can get referrals to instruction programs in your particular locale. Please remember that Natural Family Planning is reliable only if the couple are really committed and well-versed in the method. You should follow your cycles a good six months before actually using the method as your only form of birth control. And we cannot emphasize strongly enough that family planning

—both the spacing of pregnancies and contraception—
should be done with serious thought and interpersonal
communication. Learn the method thoroughly before
beginning to use it, and when doubts arise, err on the
side of caution.

Referral Sources for Instruction
in Natural Family Planning

THE HUMAN LIFE AND NATURAL
FAMILY PLANNING FOUNDATION
1511 K Street, N.W.
Washington, D.C. 20005
    (202) 393-1380

THE INTERNATIONAL FEDERATION
FOR FAMILY LIFE PROMOTION
1511 K Street, N.W.
Washington, D.C. 20005
    (202) 783-0137

SERENA CANADA
55 Parkdale
Ottawa, Ontario, K1Y 1E5, Canada
    (613) 728-6536

FAMILY LIFE PROMOTION
OF NEW YORK
P.O. Box 489
Smithtown, New York 11787
    (516) 979-7056

THE COUPLE TO COUPLE LEAGUE
P.O. Box 11084
Cincinnati, Ohio 45211
    (513) 661-7612

NEW ENGLAND NATURAL
FAMILY PLANNING
c/o Roni Molloy
95 Joe English Lane
Manchester, New Hampshire 03104
    (603) 669-5076

Index

ABOUT THE AUTHORS

CHRISTINE GARFINK is a registered nurse and nursing director at a neighborhood health center in Boston. She is also a prepared childbirth teacher who actively teaches and has experience in home deliveries. HANK PIZER is a physician's assistant at Jewish Memorial Hospital in Boston, and a painter and photographer. Chris and Hank live in Cambridge, Mass., where they share the parenting of Chris's nine-year-old daughter, Katherine. Together they have authored *The New Birth Control Program*, a book designed to teach Natural Family Planning, and *Post Partum*, a book for parents about the first year of parenting. Hank is currently working on two other books to be published shortly. Both Chris and Hank have been involved in trying to bring medical information to nonmedical people in a form that is readily understood. As Hank puts it, "Years ago I decided that it was my goal to demystify medicine and provide my knowledge in a form that anyone could understand. I wanted to help people learn about their own bodies, be able to ask the right questions of themselves and their doctors, and to speak to them in a way that allowed them to feel intelligent and competent. Too often doctors make their patients feel silly or stupid by their attitude and way of communicating. I want very much to alter that."

Chris's interest in medicine is rooted in the Woman's Self Help Movement. She says, "I want to combine medicine and feminism, and to provide women with the knowledge to understand themselves and their bodies, and to be in control of those forces. Medicine is the area in which I can exert the most effective positive influence for women."

How's Your Health?

Bantam publishes a line of informative books, written by top experts to help you toward a healthier and happier life.

ALL FOR THE FAMILY

Choose from this potpourri of titles for the information you need on the many facets of family living.

☐	12208	**THE FUTURE OF MARRIAGE** Jessie Bernard	$2.75
☐	12179	**LOVE AND SEX IN PLAIN LANGUAGE** Eric W. Johnson	$1.50
☐	12208	**THE PLEASURE BOND** Masters & Johnson	$2.50
☐	02814	**DARE TO DISCIPLINE** J. Dobson	$1.95
☐	02108	**A PARENT'S GUIDE TO CHILDREN'S READING** Nancy Larrick	$1.95
☐	11385	**P.E.T. IN ACTION** Thomas Gordon with J. Gordon Sands	$2.50
☐	12296	**THE FUTURE OF MARRIAGE** J. Bernard	$2.75
☐	10536	**THE BOYS AND GIRLS BOOK ABOUT DIVORCE** Richard A. Gardner	$1.50
☐	11378	**HOW TO GET IT TOGETHER WHEN YOUR PARENTS ARE COMING APART** Richards & Willis	$1.75
☐	11037	**WHO WILL RAISE THE CHILDREN?** James Levine	$1.95
☐	12742	**NAME YOUR BABY** Lareina Rule	$1.95
☐	11227	**YOU AND YOUR WEDDING** Winnifred Gray	$1.95
☐	11365	**OF WOMAN BORN: Motherhood as Experience and Institution** Adrienne Rich	$2.95

Buy them at your local bookstore or use this handy coupon for ordering:

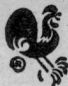

Bantam Book Catalog

Here's your up-to-the-minute listing of over 1,400 titles by your favorite authors.

This illustrated, large format catalog gives a description of each title. For your convenience, it is divided into categories in fiction and non-fiction—gothics, science fiction, westerns, mysteries, cookbooks, mysticism and occult, biographies, history, family living, health, psychology, art.

So don't delay—take advantage of this special opportunity to increase your reading pleasure.

Just send us your name and address and 50¢ (to help defray postage and handling costs).
